BEHIND THE BARS
RUTHLESS FITNESS

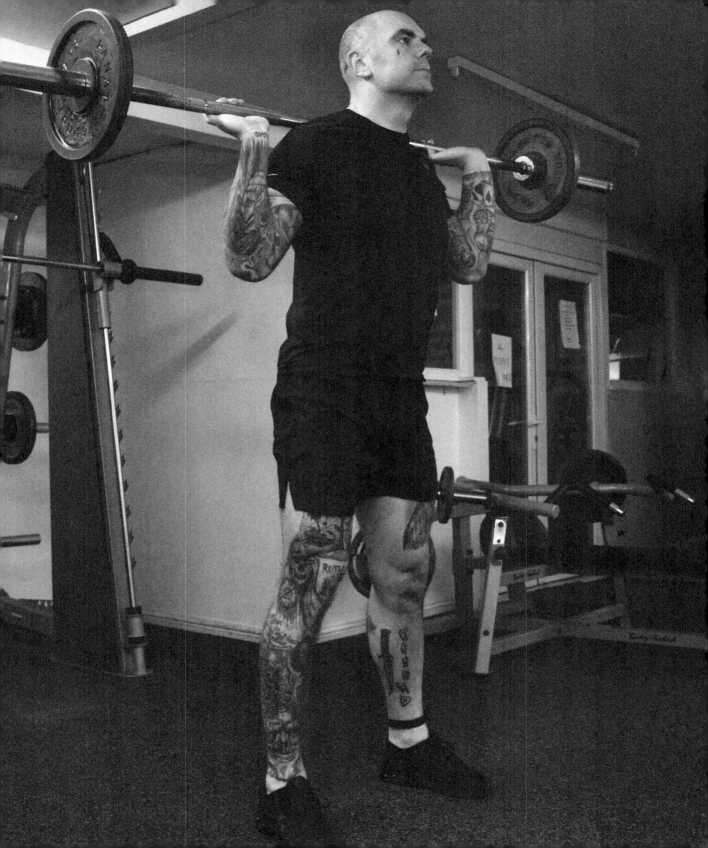

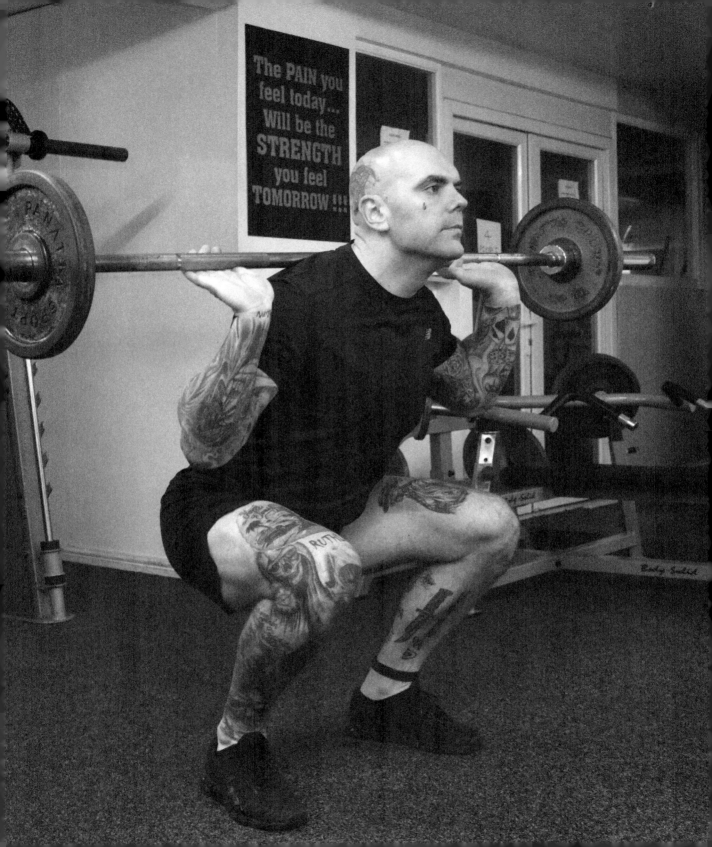

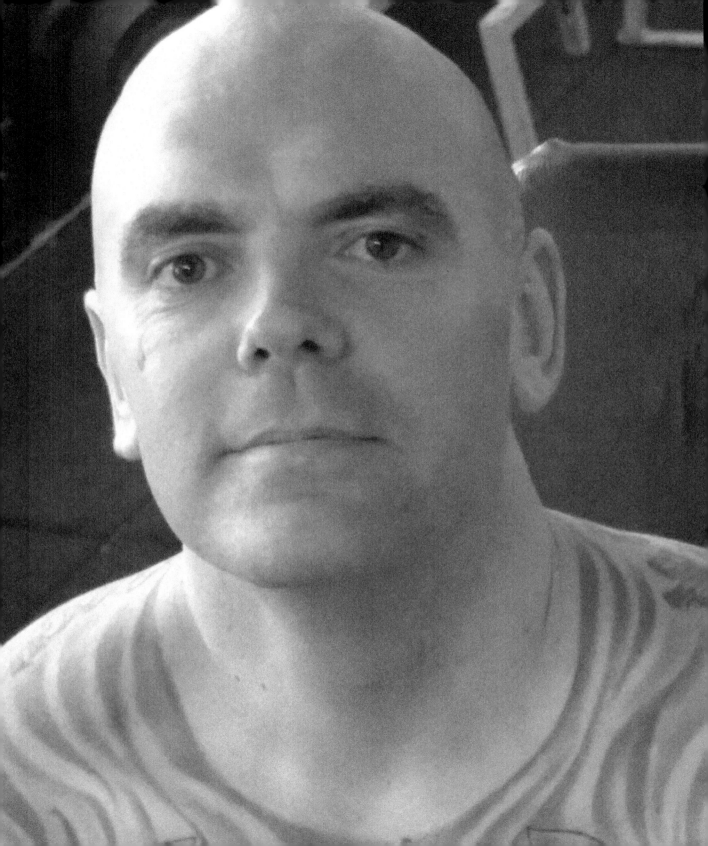

"My inspiration for writing this book came from wanting to help others who are in similar situations, people suffering with mental health and people who want to better themselves but just don't have the guidance on how to do this." - Ricky Killeen

CONTENTS

Introduction 1 - 2
What Benefits You Will See 3 - 4
About Me 5 - 8
Audience 9 - 10
Psychology 11 - 20
Nutrition 21 - 30
Body Types 33
Warming up 34
Stretching 35 - 52
Walking, Jogging, Running & Sprinting 53 - 54
Fitness Test 55 - 56
Abs Training 57 - 70
Cardiovascular Training 71 - 72
Prisoner Dumbbell Workout 73 - 74
Beginner Cell Workout 75 - 76
Yard Workout 77 - 78

Working Out In The Gym 79 - 81
Bulking Workout 82 - 83
Cutting/Getting Lean Workout 84 - 86
The SIX Month Weightlifting Cycle 87 - 88
The SIX Month Fitness Plan 89 - 96
Additional BodyWeight Circuits 97 - 98
Advanced Circuits 99 - 101
My Workout 102 - 103
Barbell Circuits 104 - 105
Additional Barbell Circuits 106 - 108
Bodyweight Exercises 109 - 148
Weight Lifting Exercises 149 - 206
Acknowledgments 207 - 208
Before & After 209 - 210
Dedication Page 211 - 212
Ruthless Fitness 213 - 214

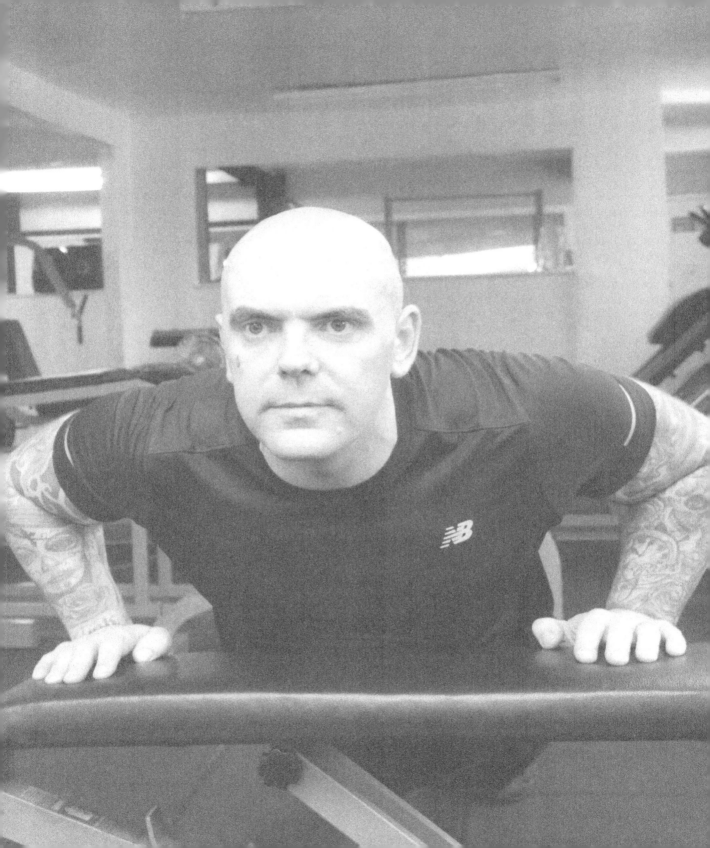

INTRODUCTION

I wrote this book to give people an insight into how to get fit and healthy in prison. Doing something positive with your time is not only going to make you feel better but it will make you look better and give you a better outlook on life. The best thing about this book, is that everything has been my reality and living proof of how to better yourself whilst getting fitter, stronger and mentally stronger. The individuals reading this book will be able to relate to what I have wrote about, as they will be experiencing similar issues. This guidance can help change your life and mindset. This advice has not come from a professional who hasn't had the life experiences, it has come from someone who has experienced prison life and know exactly what it is like to be trapped in your own thoughts in a prison community.

This book will guide you how to workout from beginner to advanced training all without the need for any equipment. This book is based around bodyweight exercises and body-building. I want to keep it as simple as possible with access to full workout routines. There are numerous books out there on fitness and nutrition but I wanted my book to be based on limited access to equipment and certain foods.

One of the main messages I want to get across in this book is to the younger generation. The message is to choose fitness as a way of life and use it to better yourself. It is better, the younger you are, when you start this way of life, training, keeping your mind occupied with workouts and being fit and healthy. Once you get in the mindset of being in good shape and feeling good about yourself it will keep you away from the negative influences in life at a young age. If you choose fitness at a young age and keep clear of the substance abuse it will set you on the path for a good life as you will be doing positive things in life and not committing crimes to pay for the substances you might be taking.

Looking back on my life I wish I had a good role model in my life to show me how to get fit, healthy and workout because it might have steered me clear of alcohol and drug use at an early age. Living on council Estates, growing up around alcohol and drug use, the majority of youngsters follow this trend and get stuck in a cycle of alcohol and drug use, but if we had more people around to help the youngsters which is what I'm trying to promote then we would have more young people living a more positive lifestyle. If we teach the younger generation to live positively and get in a positive mindset, wanting to better their lives and also promote good mental health, then we will have a lot more youngsters living pro social lives and feeling good mentally as well as physically.

I am not going to sell you the dream where you can get fit in 4 weeks with a six pack after doing 3 20 minute workouts a week because it just doesn't work like that. If you want to see the benefits you have to put the work in. Although 3 20 minute workouts a week might be a good place to start, if you are a beginner.

After 3 months of doing these workouts you are going to see some difference in your body shape, weight and fitness ability. It takes 6 months to be at your peak fitness of training every day like this but week by week you will notice a difference. As you can see by my pictures in this book I am not your typical 2% body fat men's health model. This is not what I am aiming for in this book although I may look like your typical big bald tattooed convict. Across the world the prison estate accumulates to quite a staggering amount of people and if I can get this book across to even just a small number of them and inspire people to train then it's all worth it. After only a couple of weeks you will feel better in yourself physically and mentally.

What this book consists of:

- **Cell workouts** where you can train right where you are without any equipment. This is not to be underestimated. A 20-45 minute workout non-stop on the spot is as good as being in the gym.

- **Yard workouts** which will make you feel better as it's in the fresh air. This is followed by the cell workout stage if you are confident enough to train in front of others. I hope you all feel confident enough after doing these workout routines and progress to the yard workouts. Once you start doing them, you will realise how fit you are becoming and your confidence will grow.

- **Gymnasium workouts** where you train with weights to build muscle and gain strength.

- **Mental health and the benefits** of working out. I am no mental health nurse but having suffered from anxiety and depression myself whilst in prison I know how doing these workouts and keeping the mind focused will help you feel positive.

This book is full of a wide variety of workouts but whichever one you pick they all have the desired outcome of making you feel better mentally and physically. It's just giving you a choice of what you want to achieve whether it's bulking, cutting, getting fit or getting big.

A lot of books just concentrate on one goal but this book focuses on different workouts so you can choose what's best for you. They all have the same end result to make us feel better and fitter than ever.

The best way to follow these workout routines is by getting some blank sheets of paper and a felt tip pen and writing down whichever workout you are doing on that day so you have it in front of you and take it to the gym, on the yard or wherever you workout. By writing down your workouts it's easier to follow and the circuits for example write the circuits onto separate bits of paper and write what weeks you are on so it makes it easier to follow.

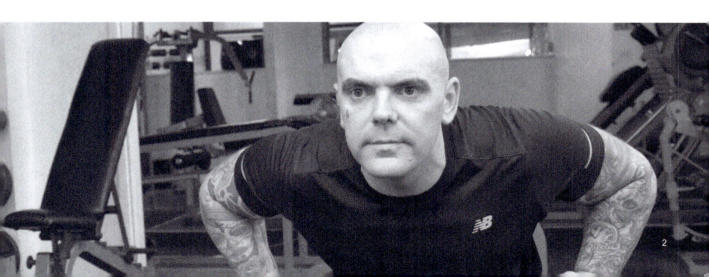

What Benefits YOU Will See:

The physical benefits you will see:

- An increase in fitness levels and strength.
- Toning of muscles and definition.
- A desire to want to workout.
- Flexibility and balance as you get used to the exercises.
- An increase in a healthy appetite.
- Your immune system will be boosted helping you fight off illnesses and diseases.
- It will also benefit your posture as your muscle strengthen up.
-

The mental benefits you will see:

- You will feel like you are achieving something and will feel much more relaxed.
- You will feel a lot more tired at night time and sleep much better.
- You will feel good about your self image as you begin to look more healthier and feel much fitter.
- You will have more confidence, feel more sociable and want to talk to other people about your workouts which in turn gives you something to talk about on Association.
- You will feel less stressed and agitated.
- After only a couple of weeks you will feel better in yourself physically and mentally.

Not being able to sleep sometimes is down to the fact we think that we are tired because our minds are exhausted but when in reality our bodies aren't tired. This is because we have not done any exercise and have been lying around all day, so what we need to do is some type of physical exercise so that not only our minds are tired, but our bodies are tired too. This in turn will help us sleep better and feel better mentally.

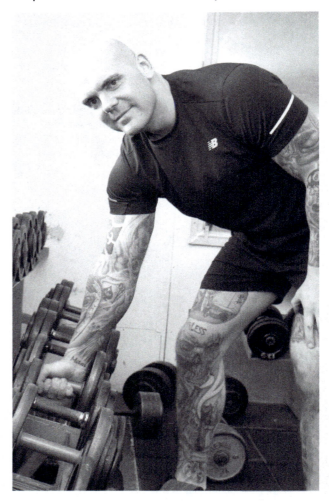

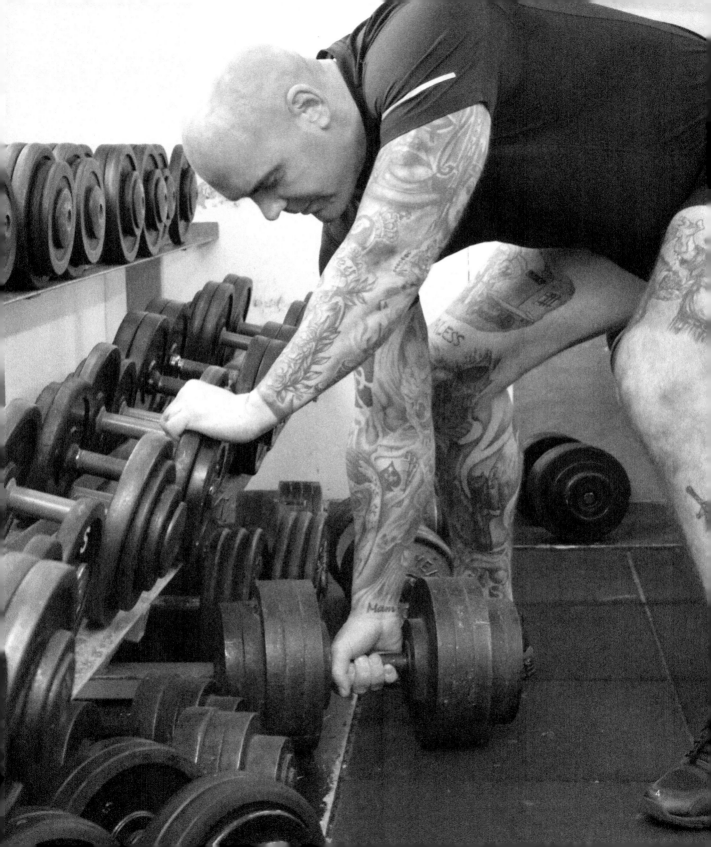

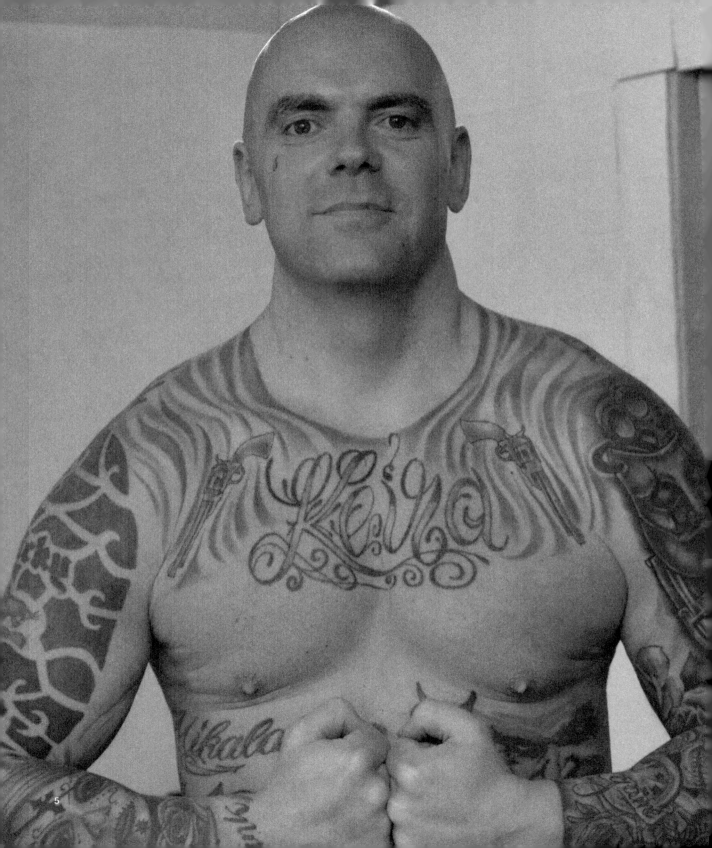

ABOUT ME

I was locked up a week before my 21st birthday. I didn't have any ambition and goals in life. I had never trained consistently, although I had done some training when I was younger, I never really stuck with it. When I arrived in Castington Young Offenders Prison I knew I wanted to join the gym and start training. I was 15 & 1/2 stone when I arrived and I aimed to get as big as I could by lifting weights. I remember the first day in the gym and I used the bench press and I attempted 60kg. I couldn't lift it. I could only lift 50kg for a couple of reps but this didn't put me off, it only made me more determined. After a couple of months I was transferred to HMP Durham men's prison. I remember going on the treadmill and jogging for seven minutes and when I got off I could see stars and felt disorientated. This was the moment when I thought "I am only 21 and so unfit" so from that moment on I quit smoking and have never smoked since.

I carried on weightlifting and doing light cardio. At the time I was training five times a week and my strength and weight started to gradually increase. During this time I was experiencing anxiety and depression but I didn't understand those feelings and what was happening to me. It wasn't until I spoke with the doctor and he explained to me that the feelings I was experiencing was panic attacks. I had a lot going on and I had never been to prison before. I had been using cocaine, ecstasy and cannabis on a regular basis. I was also drinking alcohol daily and I was facing a life sentence for a violent attack on a gang rival that I committed whilst intoxicated, something which I deeply regret. When I was training, I felt like I could escape these feelings. I focused all my energy on my training sessions and just picked up advice and workout routines from the other lads.

After six months I had gained a stone in weight and was much stronger but still didn't really have a set routine in the gym and wasn't lifting the weights correctly due to never been shown. Everyone was just trying to lift as much as possible with really bad form.

I could bench about 80kg by this point. I was sentenced to 4 years IPP, an indeterminate life sentence with a minimum tariff of four years to serve, before I could be considered for parole. My mental health was no better and I tried different types of medication to help with my anxiety and depression but to also help with the sleepless nights.

I was then transferred to HMP Frankland a maximum security prison and decided to stop taking the medication as it seemed to be making my panic attacks more intense. This is when I really started to get into my fitness and bodybuilding. I used this as a coping mechanism for my mental health problems.

It took me over 12 months before I could bench 100kg but with some advice, guidance and my determination I really started to feel much better physically and mentally. I was surrounded by men serving 30 to 40 years as well as life sentences. Some of these men had been training for 20 years and were fitness fanatics.

I started asking for different workout routines from different lads and built up my own program. I done barbell circuits for about a year and I was the fittest I had ever been. I was now 17 & 1/2 stone, benching 125kg, squatting 200kg and deadlifting 230kg. Gradually, after a couple of years my anxiety was much better. I was feeling good about myself physically and mentally.

After three years, I was transferred to HMP Acklington which is now Northumberland. I got a job as a gym orderly and I worked hard for several qualifications including gym instructor and weightlifting awards. I was released after serving five years and I was 25 years old. I was full of ambition and was a totally different person to what I was five years previous.

I had done cardio, weightlifting and circuits in that time and I had an excellent understanding of different workout programs to achieve different goals. Whether my goal was to get as big as possible, as strong as possible or as fit and as lean as possible. I had a whole new outlook on life and I was determined to be successful in life. I could have used drugs as an easy option in prison but with my determination and motivation I came out stronger and healthier, physically and mentally than I had ever been in my life.

I went on to marry my girlfriend and have four children. I have owned three businesses in the following nine years. In those 9 1/2 years I was out of prison, I have seen first hand and experienced a lot of mental health issues. My best friend since we where 10 years old committed suicide and I found him. This event impacted my mental health and still I trained and done workouts to distract my mind from the torment I was going through. My wife's aunty committed suicide only a couple of years later which affected us both very deeply, another one of my very good friends also committed suicide a couple of years later which sent my mind into turmoil. The reason I am mentioning these events in this book is to help others in similar situations. I have been at rock bottom and turned my life around. When I was having feelings of anxiety, despair and depression I picked myself up and continued to workout to help rid myself of these feelings and do something positive instead of further creating negativity. Things where going well for me and I was feeling very fit and healthy but then after being a free man without being in any trouble for 9 & 1/2 years, I found myself back in the same prison, having been recalled, experiencing the same feelings and at rock bottom knowing I had not only let myself down but now my wife and children. I was back in prison 12 months waiting for a parole hearing after being recalled.

The mental health I was experiencing in the first few months was worse than I had ever experienced before. I continued to workout to escape from these feelings and help me sleep at night. I was training four times a week in the gym lifting weights and I was benching 170kg. I was doing yard workouts 2 to 3 times a week for fitness but I made the mistake of eating the wrong foods and went up to 19 stone. Even though I was big, muscular and looked good, I was gaining fat and feeling the excess weight.

We were locked down in March 2019 because of the Coronavirus Pandemic and were on 23 hour lockdown. I made the decision to use my time getting really fit again and I lost 2.5 stone. I am now 16.6 stone and I am the fittest and healthiest I have ever been in my life. Mentally I felt so good about myself and overcame the feelings I was experiencing on my first few months back in prison. I have lived and experienced the effects of mental health and how fitness can change your mindset and make you stronger. Stronger in body and mind. I started doing circuits at the beginning of lockdown, I completed these in my cell and on the yard. This book was primarily going to focus on bodyweight exercises as that is how I have getting so fit and healthy but I wanted to share my experiences with the people sitting there in the same position I was in at 21.

I want this book to help everybody, whatever your goal is. I have trained for eight months, 6 days a week sometimes 7. Somedays I train twice a day and have Saturdays off. I was already relatively fit but it took me about 3 to 4 months of doing circuits every day to really reach my potential and feel at my peak fitness. There were times then and now when I feel like giving up with the workouts but I just remember how good I feel afterwards.

For someone who hasn't trained before it definitely takes 6 months of training to start to see how much progress you make. It takes 6 months to become super fit. Whilst I was in prison I have helped about 6 lads to better themselves and helped them get extremely fit with my workouts. I gave them advice which is all in this book.

It is living proof that what I am preaching in this book actually works, not only did it work for me it worked for the lads I was training with and giving fitness plans to. I formed some close friendships whilst I was in prison and I took pride in myself knowing that I had helped others that where struggling and in the same position I was in. The lads that I was training with all had there own personal problems and mental health issues and I talked with them aswell as been training partners. In those intense 30-45 minute workouts on the yard our minds where distracted and we where all united in getting fit and releasing our minds from the negative surroundings.

When I completed this book I was out of prison 8 months, after sitting my parole and been released on life license, I am now back home with my beautiful wife and 4 kids who I am fortunate to have. I was on GPS tagging for 6 months but I was not letting none of these barriers get in the way of achieving my goals that I have set for myself to better my life.

I am continuing to remain positive and help other people who are struggling and just need some help and guidance. In the 3 months after been released I have been nonstop typing up this book and getting it prepared. I also continued with my health and fitness and bought a load of training equipment to workout in my backyard as we were still in lockdown due to the coronavirus.

The training I am doing is still pretty much the same apart from I am lifting weights and doing barbell circuits (the ones which are in this book). I have set up my own social media accounts promoting positivity and good mental well-being which has had great feedback on what I am doing.

I am proud to say people have reached out to me for help and advice for mental health and fitness issues, it's proven that what I do does help people and that's what my goal is with this book to help others who are struggling in life which we all do at some point. It's about talking about it and what to do in these situations.

I have also set up my own clothing range called **RUTHLESS FITNESS** and it all comes together with the book as the way we train is **RUTHLESS** and if you want to better your life and get in shape you have to do it the ruthless way.

These workouts are really hard and you have to be motivated enough to push yourself to the limits. I have a lot of things in the pipeline and I am full of ambition so really busy working hard to help myself and others have a brighter future. I want to inspire people to change and better themselves because we all have potential it's just about realising what you can do and become.

It's about realising that you can change your ways, change your mindset and be a better person than you where yesterday, it's never to late and this might be the turning point in your life when the light bulb switches on and you think yes I can do this.

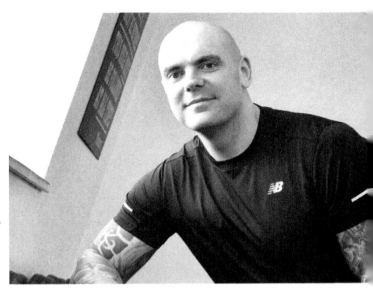

You will think I will be the person I want to be and get rid of that negative mindset and them negative emotions that are holding you back.

Look me up on social media if your getting released or if your sitting there at home wanting to escape from the past that is holding you back, I will help in any way I can.

In the back of this book I have put a list of helplines and organisations that are there to help people struggling with mental health and need someone to talk to. When we get released there just seems to be no help at all and like I mentioned I am fortunate enough to have a loving family and really close friends who I can talk to and confide in. There's huge amounts of people daily been released or sitting at home that just don't have the help or support and there's no helpful information given to us from probation or the prison which I believe every person being released should be provided with. Information like this with helpful numbers in providing help if needed and this is something which I am trying to change.

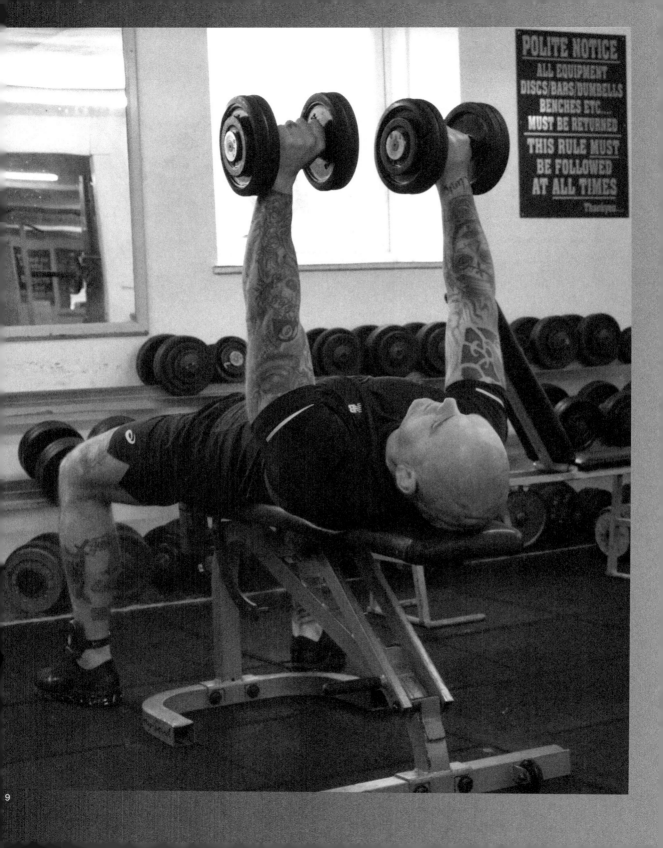

AUDIENCE

This book is for anyone of any age and sex. It can help the youngsters locked up in detention centres to the older people in their 60s who want to better themselves and improve their health and ultimately prolong their life.

The youngsters aged 15 to 21 will benefit massively as it will give them something to do and focus their mind on. It will give them a purpose in life and the younger you start the better, as you are still growing at that age. It will promote healthy bone density and structure.

This book is also aimed at anyone who is wanting to better themselves whether you are a beginner, a prisoner, suffering from mental health or just someone looking for some guidance on how to workout and do different types of training.

The reason this book is aimed at prisoners as well is because when I wrote this book I was in prison but I don't just want this to be based on prisoners training with limited equipment.

I want it to be for individuals who are sitting at home and feeling like prisoners trapped in there own thoughts. You can use this book for its workouts as a way to release from the stresses of life.

This book is also aimed at individuals who can't afford gym memberships or don't have the confidence to step foot in the gym, as well as the individuals who work and don't have enough time to go to the gym. This book could help them do a workout on their break in a car park.

This book is for everyone and it's about helping people and giving you the guidance on how to turn you into an athlete and change your mindset from negative to positive. I want to pass on the skills to help people in life which you can in turn pass on to your children and be a good role model to them.

This book is for anyone who is overweight that does not have any confidence. This book will show you how you can train in the comfort of your own cell or home until you lose weight and have the confidence to progress to working out on the yard or in the gym.

That's the beauty of this book you can do it by yourself in your own time, when you want. Although it says 3 months and 6 month plan you can taper it to your own needs and do what's best for you. Some may feel 2 workouts or circuits a week is enough and makes you feel better. Pick the workout that best suits your needs and practice it but don't get comfortable with doing easy workouts as you will not progress. Try to follow the routines as best as you can and always try and get better week by week.

It is also suited for older people because age is no barrier. I have come across some really fit men over the years some over 60. I started working out when I was 21 years old when I entered the prison system and I only wish I had started sooner as it's the best thing I have ever done.

I have trained almost every day and have hardly ever missed a week in the 14 years I have been working out. Most of the youngsters of that age just want to lift weights and get big and be as strong as possible yet they don't know how to workout properly but don't worry I will talk about that later in this book.

PSYCHOLOGY

This section is about the psychology behind working out and how it makes you feel better mentally aswell as physically. When in prison this can be the hardest place to train and workout because you have a lot going on. The stresses of prison life can affect the way we workout but believe me if you persist with it you can train through it. It becomes a way of life for you and you workout to make yourself feel better. I wrote this from my own personal experiences.

If you are having a bad day, didn't sleep properly, are on medication to keep you calm or to help you sleep this can all impact on your thoughts and the way you feel. Ultimately this could effect your workouts but by the end of the 6 month workout plan you will see these barriers that may have been preventing you from working out soon become the reason you want to workout.

The workouts help you sleep better, make you feel calm, relaxes your anxiety, stops you from feeling depressed and puts you in a positive mindset. So what you need to do is stop them negative thoughts and turn them into positive ones, for instance when we think, "I can't be bothered, I'm in a bad mood," take that negative thought which we will call a red thought and turn it into a positive thought which we will call a green thought. "I am going to workout and I know I can do this and I will feel better," it can be that easy to have a red thought and not workout. This will make you feel worse for the rest of the day so we need to flood our minds with green thoughts when these arise and continue to workout which will ultimately make us feel better.

You could even do this by writing down positive thoughts and putting them up in your cell or a good place to have positive quotes is above your toilet so when you're taking a pee you can look at it, read them and just by surrounding yourself with positivity will make you feel so much better. A good green thought is,"It's only a 30 minute workout I can do this" and a good quote I have above my toilet is, "You have to be at your strongest when you're feeling at your weakest." So by doing the green thought process we are telling our brains we can do something when we feel like not doing it.

Moving forward and battling on through the workout no matter how hard it is mentally as well as physically draining, we can overcome the negative thoughts and feel so much better once we have completed the workout. When you have completed the workout it feels like you have achieved something and your mental state all round feels that much better.

When doing physical fitness our brains release a chemical called dopamine which makes us feel so much better about ourselves, our brain also releases endorphins which trigger a positive feeling in the body which gives you that heightened feeling after a workout. Exercise also reduces stress hormones.

Determination & Motivation

This is what you are going to need loads of because without the determination to change and motivation to workout you will ultimately fail.

I'm going to give you a couple of tools to help you with this as I know from experience how hard it can be sometimes but with a little help and push from yourself you can do it.

The first tool I am going to talk about is self talk, this is something I use on a daily basis and helps me realise and achieve my goals.

An example of this is *" I can do this, it's only 45 minutes"*. A good self talk statement I use whilst I am training and feel like giving up is *"DNF,"* which means in sports competition terms, did not finish. I have tweaked this and I say to myself *" do not fail "*. I repeat to myself DNF and I think of myself failing if I don't finish the session or the circuit and guess what I have never had a **DNF (DID NOT FINISH)**.

I am a competitive person so when I am training, which is sometimes by myself I am always competing against myself and trying to beat previous times and lifts. This is what works for me. Another good tool I use which helps a lot is being assertive with myself, assertive with my attitude and thoughts around working out which helps keep me motivated.

An example of this is, *"I will do this workout and I will smash the shit out of it."* By doing this with yourself it avoids the doubts that you have experienced before you workout. The doubts about whether you can be bothered or not and by being assertive it keeps you away from them passive thoughts such as, *"I can't really be bothered with this"*.

This all links in to help keep you motivated and determined because it all comes down to how motivated and determined you are. It is so easy to have a thought that puts you off and stops you from training. You may think of your own thoughts that you could say to yourself when you are having a mental blockage that will help you along and aide you in achieving your goals.

Below is a chart to help you challenge these unhelpful thoughts with helpful thoughts just to give you some help if you ever have these thoughts.

UNHELPFUL	HELPFUL
I can't be bothered today.	I can do this. I've done it before when I've felt like this and smashed it.
I don't feel myself.	I will feel much better once I've worked out.
I haven't got the energy.	Do the best you can.
I feel like shit.	I will feel amazing when I have finished.
I'm in a bad mood.	I will be in a much better mood when I complete a workout.

Mental Health & Physical Training

Mental health affects the best of us and sometimes without even knowing it. To suffer from mental health doesn't mean that your mental or have to have been seen by a doctor and diagnosed with something.

We all suffer from it at some point and a lot of us suffer from it on a daily basis, this could be just feeling down or anxious for no apparent reason. Its about knowing how we deal with it and move on from it. The best and most positive way of doing this is by doing physical training, whether it be running, circuits, weights, cardio or a mixture of them all. By taking part and completing a workout even if we don't feel like doing it, it will make you feel so much better about yourselves afterwards.

The first step is recognising that you have a problem or a mental health issue and the best first most important thing to do is talk to someone about it. It's not something to be ashamed of and that's where the mental training part of this book comes in. It's about gathering these thoughts and feelings, understanding them and realising why these thoughts and feelings are happening. It could be the environment your in, your past experiences and your lifestyle. If your in a negative mindset and you continue to act and think in a negative way, then it is not going to achieve anything apart from further negative actions and consequences. If your wanting to change and better yourself you have to train physically and mentally. If your lifestyle is bad and negative then it will have a negative impact on your mental wellbeing and its how to change your lifestyle to better yourself. If your in an environment like prison or a bad situation at home and it's something or somewhere you don't want to be then again this will all impact on your thoughts, emotions and it's about managing them and doing something positive to get out of this situation. If you have had a traumatic past or you have had something negative happen to you at some point in your life whether it was as a child or recently (which the majority of us have) then it is going to impact on your thoughts and emotions or the way you think. What you have to do is confront these thoughts and feelings and talk about them, once you have spoken about them that is the first step to mental training and you will already begin to feel better. The next step is to think of positive things. Think of some goals you have set for yourself and think of what you want in the future and how you are going to feel when you achieve them. If you wake up thinking negative because of a rough sleep or your head is clouded because of nightmares and bad dreams then start thinking positive and think of doing something positive in your day. Think of the workout you are going to do whether it's a circuit or a walk, this will distract your mind from the negative thoughts and you will begin to feel better. It's all about training your mind to be better than it is and flooding it with positive vibes.

It's not just about doing the workouts for a few weeks it's about been motivated enough to continue working out constantly and making it a part of your life. It helps to beat stress, depression, anxiety and feelings of despair. As you progress, when you do an intense workout the heightened feeling you get afterwards is the reward for your hard work and it doesn't stop there. You will be thinking about what you're going to eat, how much your eating, what workout you will be doing the next day and where you will be doing it whether it is in your cell, at home, in the gym, on the yard or in your garden. Like I said before this is a way of life, it's about being consistent and carrying on doing something positive that is going to give you a positive outlook and mindset. Once you have been doing my workouts and have become an advanced athlete because thats ultimately what you will become, you can take the exercises and adjust the circuits and create your own plan to further your potential gains.

This could even be a basis for future employment in the fitness industry, just look at me and how far I have come, now I have wrote a book about it. Take advantage of the situation and it can be life changing, I have known lads that have gone on to become fitness instructors and personal trainers. You would have to further your education but this could be the basis for it.

There may be times in your workouts where you feel you are not improving but persevere with it and you will see the improvements. This is what you call a plateau, when you feel like you have hit a wall and you are not improving. If you feel like giving up, maybe have a couple of days to rest and recover or go back to doing more reps on the bench press with a lighter weight to build more strength. We all reach this point but believe me, when you stick with it and get past it you will feel incredible.

Another important factor to remember it's not about competing with other people, it's about competing against yourself and getting fitter. If you look at other people training and think they are quicker, can perform reps faster, lift more weight then thinking like this will put you off and stop you from achieving your own personal goals. It's not about the other person, it's all about you and what you can achieve that you never thought was possible.

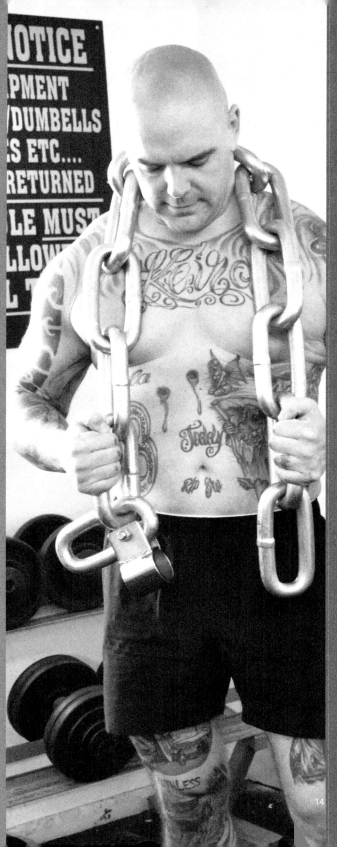

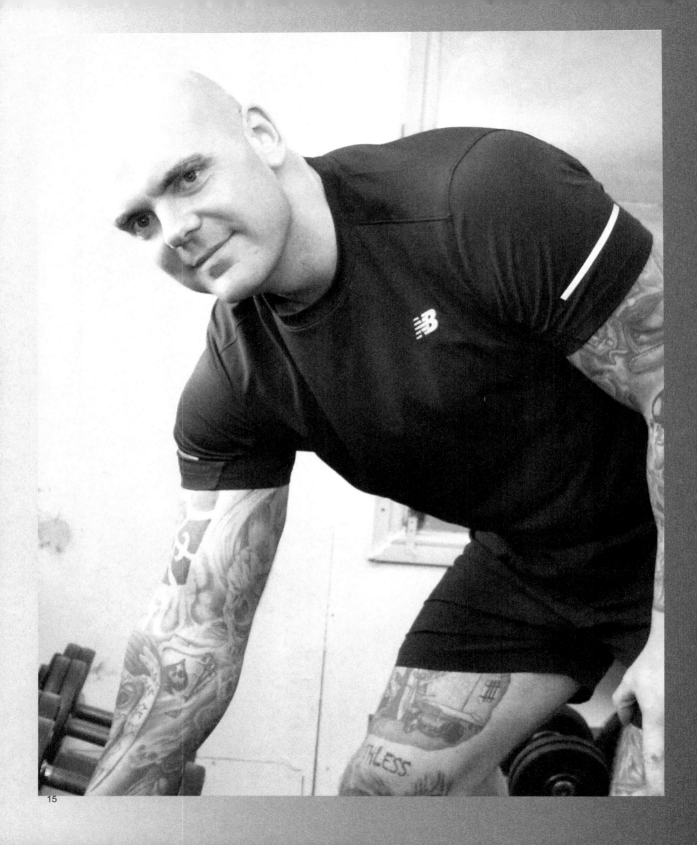

Positive & Inspiring Quotes

"We have to be at our strongest when we are feeling at our weakest"

"Train hard, eat well = feel good"

"Be stronger than you were yesterday"

"Set some goals, stay quiet about them, smash the shit out of them and be proud of yourself"

"Stop worrying about what other people think of you and dont dwell on the past"

"Never Give up, it is NOT an option"

"The more time you spend on regret, the more you beat yourself up and it stops you doing something good with the rest of your life"

"Be strong now because things will get better, it may be cloudy now but it won't be clouded forever"

"A healthy body and a healthy mind is all you need"

"When you build strength in silence, people dont know what to attack"

"Dont judge yourself by your past, its in the past and you don't live there anymore"

"I know I can do this, Im stronger than i think"

"Determination, positivity and motivation is all i need to see me through this"

"Never let a bad situation bring out the worst in you, always be strong and choose to be positive"

"Make the rest of your life, the best of your life"

Improving Your Self Image

I thought I would talk about self image in my book as it's an important part of why we workout as well as getting fit. We want to look better and feel better. Like I mentioned before this book is not just about the workouts it's an all-rounder, promoting healthy living and a healthy mindset which the majority of us suffer from. It's about promoting positivity and making us feel better about ourselves. You will find as you get fitter and stronger your mind will become healthier, more focused and more positive. It may even help some of you stop using drugs. These workouts and routines will become your drug of choice. It will be the best decision you've ever made. You'll feel better about yourselves and will soon be getting compliments of people, officers, friends and family, and in turn it will create better relationships. What better way to do it and it doesn't cost anything to workout. It will make you feel better than you've ever felt in years. It improves your self image by first of all boosting your confidence and by the way you look. Once you get yourself fit and lose weight, gain weight or tone up you will look good and feel good, which in turn improves your self image.

Low Self-Esteem & Paranoia

I wanted to mention low self-esteem in this book because we are all conscious about how we look and how we think other people look at us. This creates a barrier and stops you from wanting to workout in front of others because we are worrying about what other people are thinking. We get paranoid that people are watching us as we workout. The best advice I can give is stop worrying about what other people think of you, the more you worry about other people's thoughts the more it will hold you back from achieving your goals. Working out will boost your self-esteem and you will see after a few weeks of training you won't be worrying as much, you will forget about your worries and really start enjoying your workouts.

You have to value yourself and know your worth to be able to progress first of all. Once you value yourself, you will then begin to build confidence and feel good about yourself. When you start your workout routine you will feel like you are better than what you thought of yourself and you do have the ability to be a better person. A fitter, healthier, more positive and determined person of your former self.

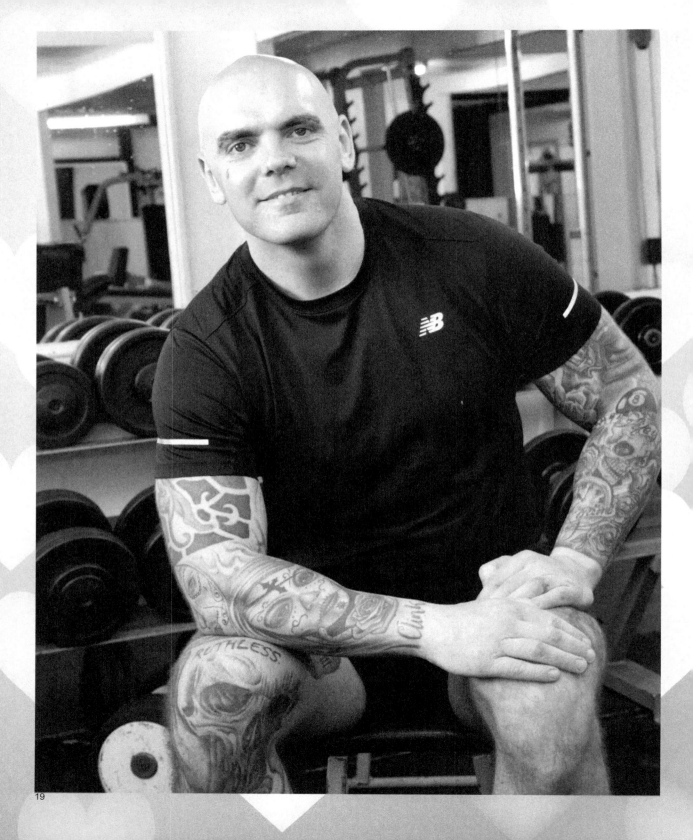

Promoting Healthy Relationships

This book also promotes healthy relationships as it gives the individual confidence and gives you something to talk about with your friends and loved ones. You won't believe the impact it has on them back home when they see you looking fitter and healthier than ever. I always say make the most out of a bad situation. It's hard enough on our loved ones back home, with us being in prison but seeing the joy on their faces and the sound in their voices when you speak to them on the phone, when they hear you are looking after your self, not dwelling on things and using drugs as a lot of people do in prison.

You could even inspire your friends, family and children to do the same and it gives you all something in common. It promotes healthy relationships among inmates when you are working out together, talking amongst yourselves helping and supporting each other along the way.

NUTRITION

In this chapter I am going to talk about what we eat and the best things to eat in prison. We all know the food we eat in prison is designed to fill you up or it is supposed to. Let's face it most the time it is a load of crap, but we can make the most of it and eat quite healthy with the choices we have.

The way I eat, I don't call it a diet because that sounds like a chore, I call it a healthy lifestyle or healthy eating. If some of us have the luxury of buying our own canteen then that's a bonus and I will tell you the best products to buy.

So as we all know we all have different body shapes and sizes and we will all have different amounts of food we need to eat. Some may be very skinny and will need to eat more calories as well as carbohydrates to gain lean muscle. Some may be very large who want to lose weight and show lean muscle, so will have to eat less carbohydrates and calories. We all want the same end result to be fit and healthy we just need to know how to eat as good as we can with what we have whilst in prison.

The standard daily calorie intake for women is 2000 calories per day and 2500 calories per day for men. I know it is hard to track calories whilst we are in prison and eating prison food as we don't know what's in it but I will try my best to advise you and guide you as best as I can.

For those of you that can buy your own food it's a lot easier to keep track of what you eat and the calories in your food. Your food is made up of what is called **macronutrients**. There are three macronutrients which is **protein, carbohydrates and fats.** Protein is what we need to build and maintain muscle, an example of this is milk, eggs, chicken, tuna.

Carbohydrates is where you get your energy from, you also get it from fats but most of your energy comes from carbohydrates. Carbohydrates can come in two forms good form and bad form in simple terms. An example of this is good carbohydrates are rice, pasta, preferably brown and from fruit and vegetables. Bad carbohydrates come from sugary foods and fried foods, examples of this are, cakes, crisps, biscuits, fries and chips.

The last macronutrient is fats. Again, I will keep it in simple terms and call this good fats and bad fats. Good fats include monounsaturated and polyunsaturated fats. Bad ones include industrial-made trans fats. Saturated fats fall somewhere in the middle. We need fat in our diet it's just we need healthy fats which comes from, nuts, fish, and the bad fats come from fried foods like fries, chips, greasy foods and margarine.

Naturally fatty fish like salmon, mackerel, sardines, tuna are good sources of omega-3 fatty acids. These are "good" fats that help keep your heart healthy. They may also help keep your brain sharp, especially as you get older.

Foods not to eat: *crisps, sweets, chocolate, fries, biscuits and fat greasy foods like sausages/ burgers.*

All of these macros end up making up our total calories for the day so it's about getting the right balance. If you are a female and your aim is to lose weight you need to eat less than 2000 calories a day. This is called a calorie deficit so you should maybe aim for around 1500 calories a day. A good way to do this is cut down on your carbohydrates and fat if you eat sugary foods like sweets crisps and cakes, cut them out and replace them with fruit and vegetables to get your carbs. For males you should be aiming for around 2000 calories a day if your aim is to lose weight. If your aim is to stay the same size then you should be eating 2500 to 3000 calories a day to maintain your size but again it has to be from healthy foods.

If you want to gain size and muscle you should up your calorie intake but again this has to be from good food sources to maintain a healthy balanced diet. Women should be eating over 2000 calories and over 3000 for men. A good way of increasing your calorie intake in prison is by eating more oats which is relatively cheap to buy on canteen, by eating a larger portion of rice or pasta from the servery which is the prison food.

Of all the macronutrients we should eat plenty of protein to maintain a healthy diet and keep lean muscle mass. The best sources of protein are tinned fish such as tuna, mackerel, sardines and peanuts. Peanut butter is a good source of protein, fats and carbohydrates. Chicken legs or even better chicken breast is also a good source of protein.

Here is a list of what I will call healthy foods which is available from the servery (prison food) :

- *Cornflakes*
- *Oats*
- *Rice crispies*
- *Muesli*
- *Chicken*
- *Chicken casserole*
- *Bean goulash*
- *Vegetable casserole*
- *Tofu and pepper wrap*
- *Salad*
- *Eggs*
- *Omelette*
- *Sag aloo*

Basically anything that is not fried, has plenty of vegetables in, always get the vegetable option and try to avoid white bread as white bread just goes straight to your stomach. I am not saying starve yourself if you don't have an option then obviously you have to eat what is given to you, but what I am saying is try to make the most of it and eat healthy if you can as it will help your progress. It will aid in building lean muscle and make you feel good overall. Always pick the fruit option from the servery instead of the dessert option like cake and custard as getting your fruit is an essential part of your nutrition for all round health benefits.

The best foods to buy from the prison canteen shop if possible are:

- *Fresh fruit and vegetables.*
- *Tinned vegetables eg, spinach, chickpeas butter beans, okra,*
    sweetcorn, beans, peas.
- *Tinned fish; Tuna, Mackerel, Sardines, Pilchards, Salmon.*
- *Eggs*
- *Tomatoes*
- *Milk*
- *Nuts*
- *Peanut butter*
- *Oats*
- *Protein powders*
- *Couscous*
- *Rice*
- *Pasta*
- *Seeds*

My Daily Meal Plan

So for me personally, a typical day of eating consists of breakfast 50g of oats, spoonful of sunflower seeds, banana, peanut butter, and milk which is a good start to the day. If this is not available I would have a bowl of cornflakes. Then at lunch time I will have a tin of mixed vegetables with a tin of mackerel and 100g of couscous. A snack in the afternoon of peanuts and a protein shake. Teatime meal I would have a small portion of rice and a healthy option from the servery like chicken casserole and vegetables. At night time I would have a protein shake or a glass of milk and a piece of fruit or whatever healthy snack I have available.

I always buy multivitamins which are an ideal nutritional supplement to go alongside your food to get some additional nutrients in your system.

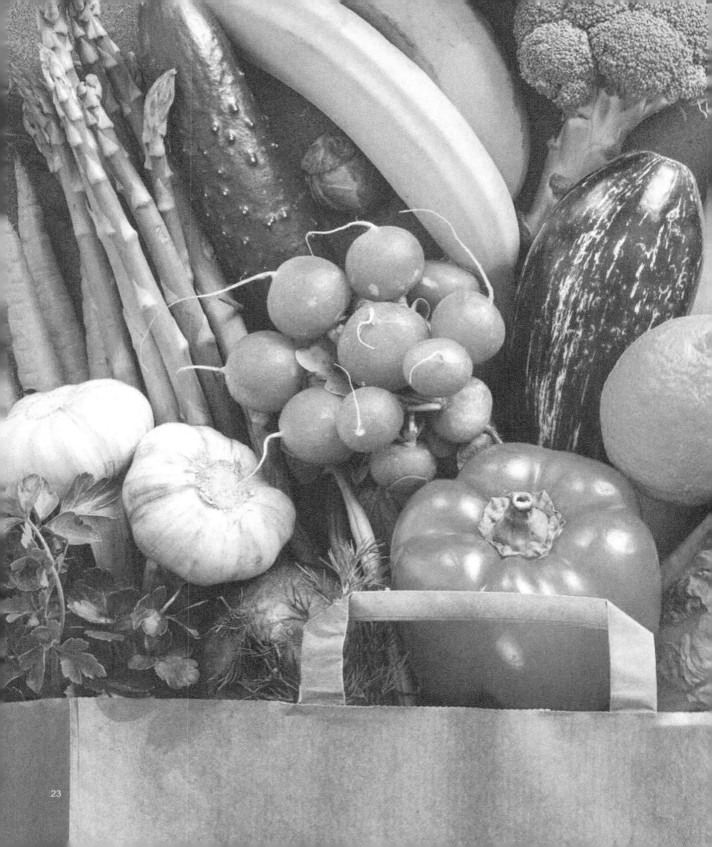

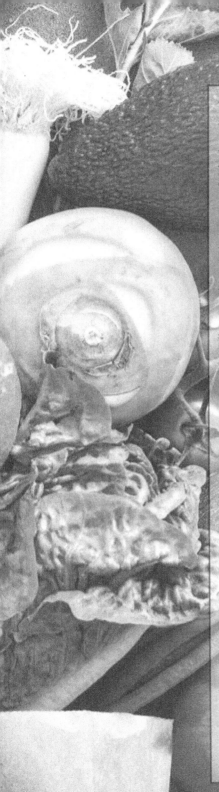

This chapter is just as a guide as I am no nutritionist or expert I am just giving you the best information to my knowledge and what has worked for me over the years. We have to do the best we can, with what we have, as being in prison we have limited options of what we can eat and it's pointing people in the right direction of eating to the best of our ability.

If your aim is to gain more weight a cheap and easy way is to increase your intake of oats, 100g of oats contains approximately 370 calories, 56g of carbs, 12g of protein and 8g of good fats which is a good balance of macros. 100g of oats is easily measured by using the small blue or grey plastic cups which we all have access to. A full cup is 100g.

For people in the community it is so much better the choice of food we can eat and also a lot cheaper. Most of the leading supermarkets have good deals on the food and we can pick food up relatively cheap. People think to eat healthy it costs more money when in fact it is actually cheaper. The best foods to buy are fresh fruits and vegetables or the frozen option is just as good and sometimes better as there is no waste and you just use what you need for that day. Frozen vegetables is just as nutritious as fresh vegetables and the same goes for canned vegetables.

A lot of us think it isn't as nutritious but it's been proven that it is just as good and sometimes cheaper. It's about what you prefer and what you can afford. Chicken fillets are the best and most affordable source of protein to buy and are cheap. They also go with almost any meal. Tinned fish is really cheap from the supermarket and can be bought for 50p a tin.

When it comes to carbohydrates it's always best to get the Brown option as it's healthier for you. Examples of this are brown rice and brown pasta as it's made from wholemeal, same goes for bread, I prefer the seeded batch which is even better.

Low fat yogurts are a good source of calcium and protein to maintain a healthy diet. Nuts are an important part of a healthy diet and have numerous health benefits but try to stay away from salted nuts and go for the raw form.

Cereals are a healthy snack but stay away from the sugary ones. Cereals like oats granola cornflakes and bran-flakes are the best ones.

SUPPLEMENTS

I have used supplements ever since I started working out and yes I really do rate them. They definitely do make a difference. The first most important one is protein.

PROTEIN

Protein intake should primarily come from whole food sources but to increase your intake it is ideal to have a couple of protein shakes throughout the day. The majority of it is affordable and there are some affordable suppliers around. Protein shakes are best taken after a workout and in between meals as a quick source of protein. It is suggested that people that workout need between 1.2 and 1.7 grams of protein per kilogram of bodyweight. Research also suggests that your body can only consume so much protein at a time. Its about 30 gram of protein at a time so should be divided up throughout the day.

CREATINE

Creatine is something I have always used and I do rate it. You will notice the difference after a couple of weeks as it enhances your progress and helps to increase your strength. It can increase lean muscle mass and help the muscles recover more quickly during exercise. It can also help with energy levels during exercise. You only need to use 5 gram of creatine per day.

I wanted to mention these two supplements because they have worked for me over the years and are the most important ones in my opinion. As you progress and can afford more supplements, I use the all in one supplements when I am in the community and they are an excellent help for strength gains. They include all the bodybuilding ingredients you need. Alongside protein and creatine they include glutamine, HMB, and amino acids. The best ones I use are Cyclone from Maxi muscle and Muscle Fuel Anabolic from USN. These two are amazing in helping gain size, strength and are worth the money.

WATER

Another vital part of a healthy living lifestyle is water. Water intake is easily accessible by everyone in the UK and is widely neglected. It is essential to keep hydrated and drink plenty of water as it aids in digestive support, it stops you from feeling tired and fatigued. You should be drinking at least 3L of water a day, this can include juice, cups of tea and coffee as it's mainly made up of water. Alongside your cups of tea you should be drinking just water.

Personally, I only have 1 cup of coffee a day with my breakfast and two protein shakes throughout the day and the rest I drink only water. A plastic cup is about 250ml so 4 of these is 1L and I have maybe 2 cups as soon as I wake up to flush my system. It also stops you from feeling as hungry. A good way to tell if you're drinking enough water is when you go to the toilet your urine will be clear.

MEALS & RECIPES

Now that I have told you what is the best foods to buy from the canteen I am going to tell you the meals that I make from this selection that is nutritious and healthy and also very tasty.

I will tell you the ingredients and how to make them. Most of the meals I make consist of spices which is what makes them so tasty, but don't worry if you don't like spicy food just don't add chili and it won't be hot. If you don't have access to a microwave you will have to use your kettle. I think the majority of you will be familiar with kettle curries etc, just be sure to keep stirring so it doesn't stick.

Most of the meals consist of tuna or other tinned fish as we can't buy much meat products on the canteen but the tuna is an ideal source of protein. A lot of the time, I just use couscous in my meals as it's cheap at £1 a pack for 500g and will get 5 meals out of it if you have 100g per serving. Couscous is made from wheat and gluten and is low in fat but high in carbohydrates, good carbohydrates and protein.

Each 100g has 354cal, 2.2g of fat, 70g of carbs and 13.6g of protein. These meals are ideal for vegans and vegetarians as well as you just have to make them without the meat or fish and just have veggie based meals. One of my all-time favourite meals used to be tuna and noodles with hot sauce but I changed this to couscous as noodles have 12 g of fat per packet, not as much protein and carbs but it is not to be dismissed as I used to eat this twice a day when I was bulking.

When cooking the following meals if you don't like tuna or tinned fish you can use tinned meat instead like chopped pork or whatever is available to you and whatever you prefer. Or if you're a vegetarian or vegan just don't add the meat or tinned fish and it is then a vegetarian meal.

Spinach & Chickpea Curry

Ingredients: half tin of spinach, half a tin of chickpeas, 1 onion, 1 pepper, 1 garlic clove, all purpose seasoning, hot curry powder, chilli powder, 100g of couscous, tin of tuna, 1 butter portion.

Method: chop onion, garlic and pepper, fry onion and garlic in kettle or microwave with butter portion for 5 minutes, add pepper and add half a teaspoon of all purpose seasoning, one heaped spoon of curry
powder, a sprinkle of chilli powder if you like it hot and mix it up, add a half a cup of water and bring to boil, then add a tin of tuna if you wish and stir, add the spinach and chickpeas and boil for a further 5 minutes add more water if needed. Put 100g of couscous in a separate bowl and cover with boiling water and leave for 3 minutes, pour Curry over couscous and enjoy.

Hot & Spicy Soup

Ingredients: Tuna, 1/3 of a tin of sweetcorn, chicken oxo cube, chili powder, jerk seasoning, half an onion.

Method: chop onion up and put in kettle or microwave bowl, add 250ml or 1 cup of water and boil, add oxo cube, sprinkle of chilli, teaspoon of Jerk seasoning and stir, add a tin of tuna and 1/3 of a tin of sweetcorn and boil for further 5 minutes. Enjoy.

Tikka Masala Couscous

Ingredients: half a tin of chick peas, 1 onion, 1 pepper, 1 garlic clove, tomato, tin of tuna, 100g couscous, all purpose seasoning, 4 in 1 Indian spices. You can use any 4 but I prefer the tikka masala.

Method: Chop onion, garlic, tomato and pepper up and boil in 250ml of water for 5 minutes, add 1 spoon of all purpose season and just over half a spoon of tikka masala and stir, add chilli if you want, add tuna and half a tin of chick peas and boil for a further 5 minutes. Put 100g of couscous in a bowl without water, pour the contents of the kettle over it, mix it up, cover and leave for 3 minutes. Enjoy.

Tomato, Chick Peas & Eggs

Ingredients: half tin of tomatoes, half a tin of chick peas and 2 boiled eggs.

Method: Pour tomatoes and chick peas in kettle or microwave and boil once. Pour into a bowl and chop 2 boiled eggs up and add to bowl, season with salt and pepper and enjoy. This is a healthy nutritious snack.

Tuna or Chicken Curry

Ingredients: tuna, 1 pepper, cooked chicken leg or breast, 1 onion, 1 pepper, 1 garlic clove, 2 tomatoes or half a tin of tomatoes 1 pack of microwave rice Maykway Curry powder.

Method: chop onion, pepper, garlic and fry in a kettle for 5 minutes. Add half a tin of tomatoes or add 2 chopped tomatoes and boil for further 5 minutes add 2 spoons of Curry powder and stir. Add a tin of tuna or a cooked chicken leg stripped and must be still warm from servery. Add water if needed if too thick boil for further 5 minutes. Cook microwave rice in microwave or empty into a see through Tea pack bag and place in a separate kettle and boil, leave for 5 minutes. Empty rice into a bowl pour Curry on top and enjoy.

Tuna or Mackerel Wraps

Ingredients: 1 onion, 1 pepper, 1 garlic clove, tortilla wraps, tin of fish, all purpose seasoning, chilli and jerk. Salad cream.

Method: Chop onion, pepper and garlic and fry in kettle with one butter portion add half spoon of all purpose sprinkle of chilli and half a teaspoon of jerk or piri piri seasoning and stir together until softened. Empty tuna onto tortilla wrap add the peppers and onions on to the top of the tuna put some salad cream on and wrap it up and enjoy.

Tuna/Mackerel/Salmon Salad Wrap

Ingredients: 1 tomato, cucumber, lettuce, peppers, onion, tin of fish, tortilla wraps.

Method: chop salad up and mix in a bowl with a tin of fish and empty onto a wrap add salt and pepper salad cream or mayonnaise and wrap it up. Enjoy.

Peanut Butter Porridge

Ingredients: peanut butter, oats, raisins, milk, banana and honey.

Method: put 100g of porridge a handful of raisins in a bowl cover with milk and leave overnight so it is soft and fluffy in the morning. Add a spoonful of peanut butter and mix, add a chopped banana and cover with honey. This is a good healthy meal but is high in calories so if you are dieting just don't put as much oats in. This is about 800 calories.

Flapjack Fruit Bowl

Ingredients: banana, kiwi fruit, yogurt, flap jack.

Method: chop up 1 banana and one Kiwi fruit and put in a bowl sprinkle in a flapjack or you can use granola put in a yoghurt or 2 of your choice and mix it up and enjoy.

Tuna & Sweetcorn Pasta

Ingredients: pasta, half a tin of sweetcorn, tuna and mayonnaise.

Method: boil 100g of pasta in a kettle for 20 minutes or until soft, put into a bowl mix half tin of sweetcorn and a tin of tuna in the bowl and add mayonnaise or salad cream.

Tuna & Pepper Pasta

Ingredients: tin of any fish, 1 pepper, 1 onion and pasta.

Method: chop onion and peppers. Cook 100g of pasta in kettle for 20 minutes or until soft. Mix peppers, onions, fish and pasta in a bowl with mayonnaise or salad cream, add salt and pepper and enjoy.

Tuna Pasta

Ingredients: pasta, 1 onion, 1 pepper, 1 garlic clove, tin of tuna, 2 tomatoes, chilli powder, all purpose seasoning and jerk.

Method: chop onion, pepper and garlic, fry in kettle or microwave in bowl for 5 minutes, add 1 teaspoon of all purpose seasoning, 1 teaspoon of jerk seasoning and 1/4 teaspoon of chilli. Stir then add 2 chopped tomatoes and boil for 10 minutes with lid on, add the tuna and stir, boil for further 5 minutes. Add the contents to 100g of cooked pasta stir and enjoy.

Couscous Mix

Ingredients: couscous, half an onion, half pepper, one egg, half a tin of chick peas, handful of peanuts and raisins, hot curry powder and 1 tin of tuna.

Method: put 100g of couscous in a bowl add a sprinkle of hot curry powder and cover with water. Finely chop onion, pepper and egg. Add to the couscous and mix it up, finally add peanuts raisins, chick peas and tuna, mix it all up and enjoy.

Korma (curry)

Ingredients: Couscous or rice, 1 onion, 1 garlic clove, 1 pepper, 1/3 of a coconut block, tin of tuna, Maykway curry powder.

Method: fry onion and pepper in kettle with garlic for 5 minutes or until softened, add 250ml or 1 cup of water and boil, add 2 teaspoons of Maykway Curry powder and stir, add 1/3 of a coconut block and let it melt and stir, add tuna, boil and stir again leave for five minutes. Put 100g of couscous in a bowl and cover with boiling water and leave to cook for 3 minutes or use a packet of microwave rice, if you have access to a microwave use it if not empty the rice into a see through tea pack bag and place in a kettle with water in, boil and leave in kettle for 5 minutes, boil again and leave for further 5 minutes, put in a bowl and pour the Curry on top of your rice or couscous. Enjoy.

Mackerel & Veg Couscous

Ingredients: Tin of mackerel in tomato sauce, 100g of couscous, tin of mixed vegetables and curry powder.

Method: put 100g of couscous in a bowl with a sprinkle of curry powder and cover with boiling water and leave for 3 minutes. Put tin of mixed veg in kettle or microwave and boil or cook for 3 minutes, drain the water and mix it in with the couscous, add the tin of mackerel and mix it all up.

Tuna Couscous

Ingredients: 1 tin of tuna, 100g of couscous, half a tin of chick peas, and 1 chicken oxo cube.

Method: put 100g of couscous in a bowl, sprinkle in 1 oxo cube and add half a tin of chick peas, pour boiling water over the top covering the couscous and chick peas (it may seem like too much water but it's best this way so it is still moist when you eat it and not dry). Cover and leave for 5 minutes, add tuna and mix it up. Enjoy (If you like hot and spicy food add a splash of hot pepper sauce).

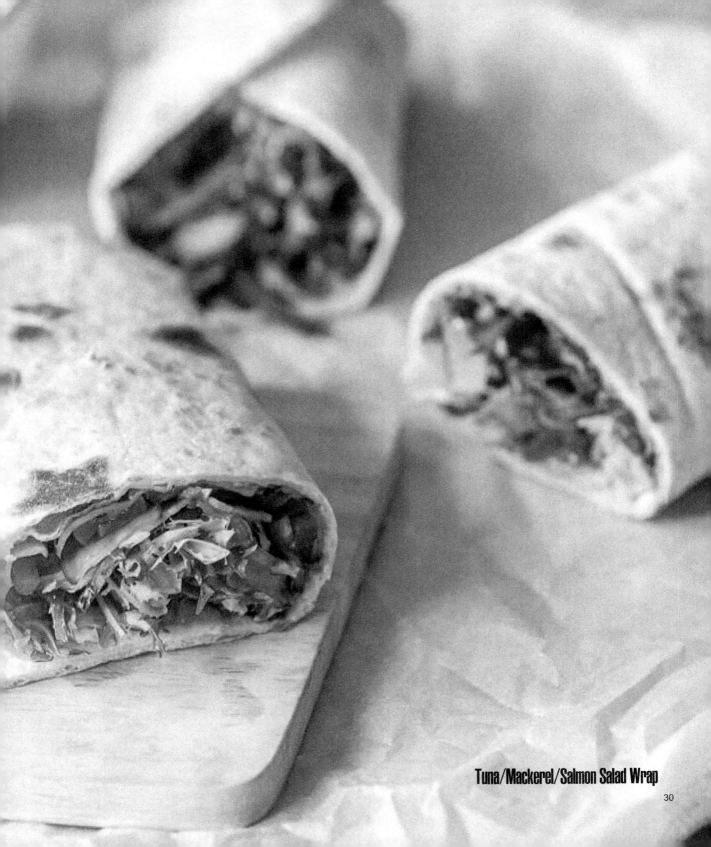

Tuna/Mackerel/Salmon Salad Wrap

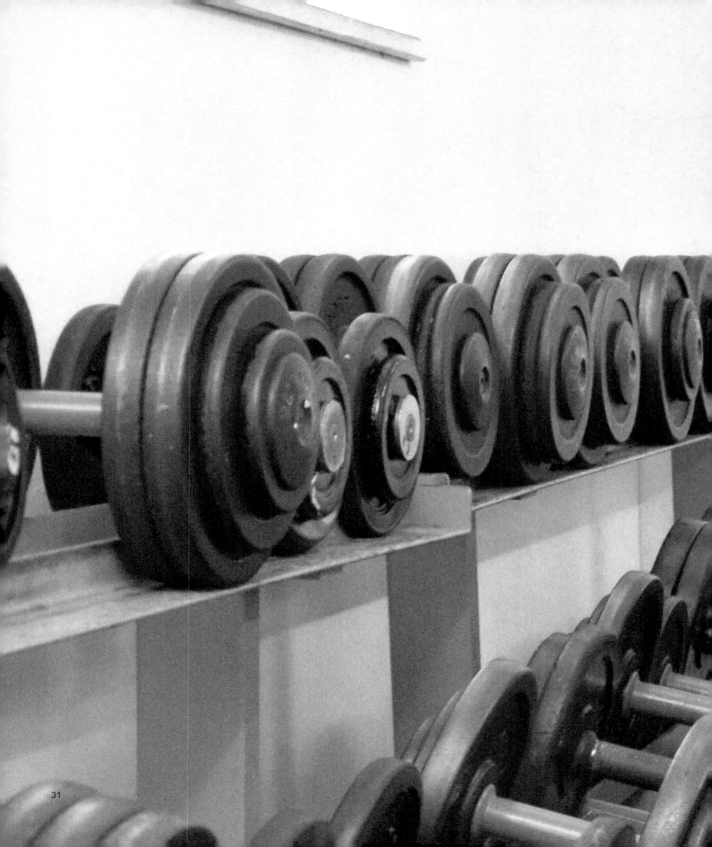

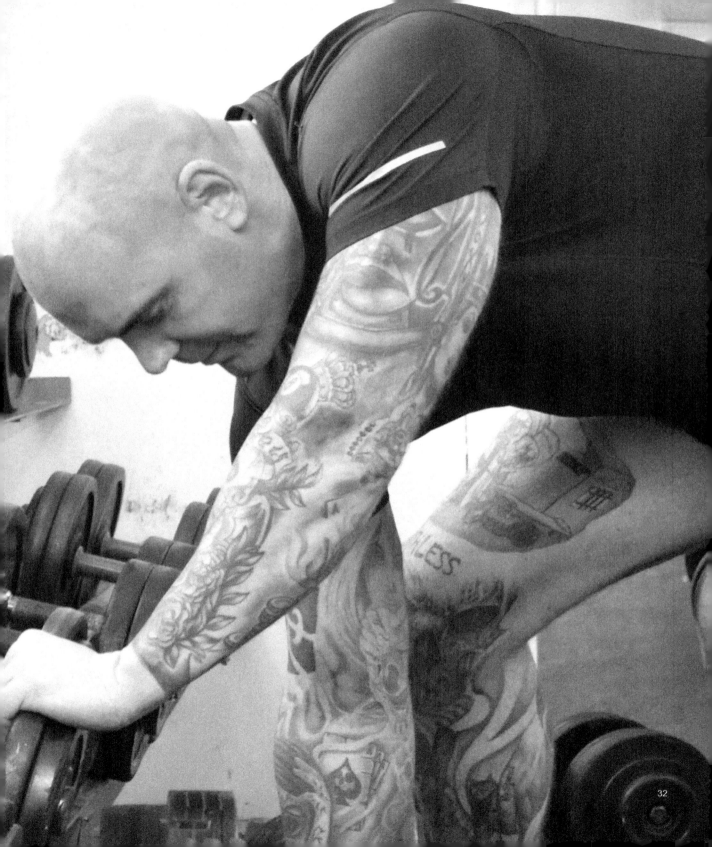

BODY TYPES

There are three different body types and we can all relate to one:

Ectomorphs - have little body fat and they are naturally thin and find it hard to gain weight.

Mesomorphs - are athletic looking, naturally lean and muscular.

Endomorphs - are quite big and round and prone to high fat storage and have trouble losing weight.

Depending on your body type you may find the workouts easier or harder but don't let this be a barrier as we are all capable of doing these workouts but some of us might be better suited to them.

WARMING UP

It is always important to warm up properly before any type of training. This is to prevent injury and also get your body ready for the workout ahead. As you do your exercises to warm up your heart starts to pump more blood around your body and begins to beat faster. Your muscles and joints will also become more mobile.

This is what a typical warmup consists of and should be done at the start of every session or workout for at least five minutes:

Five minutes light jog on the spot whilst shaking your arms out in front of you and lifting them up punching into the air as though you are shadowboxing.

10 half squats

10 press ups

10 jumping jacks

10 high knees

5 burpees

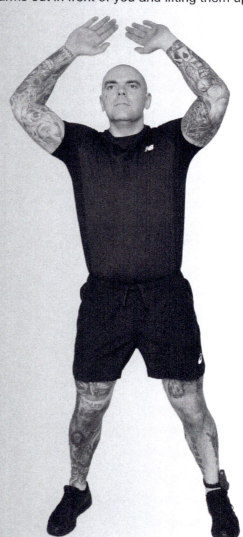

STRETCHING

Stretching is an important part of maintaining a healthy lifestyle as you need to keep your muscles and joints flexible so you can do physical exercise.

Stretching promotes flexibility and helps your joints maintain a healthy range of motion. Stretching can be really relaxing aswel if you concentrate on your breathing when you are stretching. (Take long deep breaths whilst stretching and just relax your mind and think of positive thoughts). It stops you from becoming stiff from sitting around all day. I have put stretching in the 6 months fitness plan but should be done at least 3 times a week to maintain mobility. You should always be warmed up before stretching to avoid injury as if you try to stretch when you are really stiff from lack of exercise you will end up injuring yourself. Some people believe you should stretch before working out, you can stretch before exercise but just moderately to avoid injury this is called Dynamic stretching.

Dynamic stretches are meant to get the body moving. The stretches aren't held for long. Do the stretches for a total of 5-10 minutes until your muscles and joints have loosened up. Do each stretch for at least 60 seconds having short rests every 10 seconds or so.

Dynamic stretches for warming up:

- Arm circles
- Hip rotations
- Leg swings
- Spinal rotations
- Neck circles

You can stretch after a workout to help your muscles loosen up. This is called Static stretching when you hold the stretch for at least 15 seconds. The way I do it is I stretch about 3 times a week for upto 45 minutes or until I feel flexible enough and my joints are loosened up.

You should always warm up first so for 5 minutes just jog on the spot then do the dynamic stretches first to loosen up.. Once you are warmed up you should be holding each stretch for 30 seconds. I repeat each stretch 2-3 times. If it's uncomfortable just hold for a shorter period and build up as you become more flexible. If any of the stretches cause you pain then stop doing them.

Static stretches:

- Overhead tricep stretch
- Shoulder stretch
- Reverse shoulders
- Neck flexion up and down
- Cobra pose
- Hamstring stretch
- Calf stretch
- Standing quads stretch
- Forward bending stretch
- Groin stretch
- Cat and dog stretch
- Pec and bicep stretch

ARM CIRCLES

Step 1: Stand upright facing forward.

Step 2: Lift your arms out to shoulder height.

Step 3: Start making circular motions with your arms for up to 2 minutes with short rests every 10 seconds.

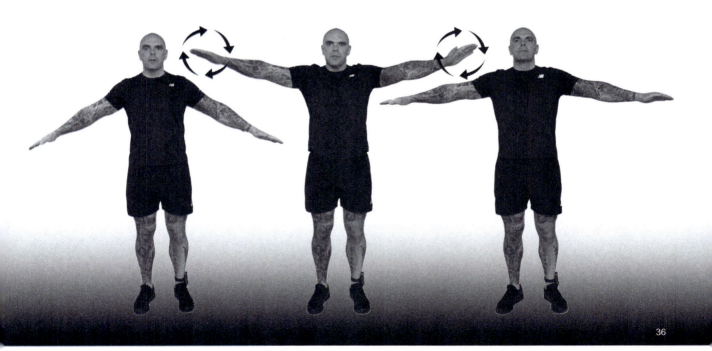

HIP ROTATIONS

Step 1: Stand with feet hip width apart.

Step 2: Pace your hands on your hips.

Step 3: Start rotating your hips in a circular motion alternating directions for a minute or two, having short rests every 10 seconds.

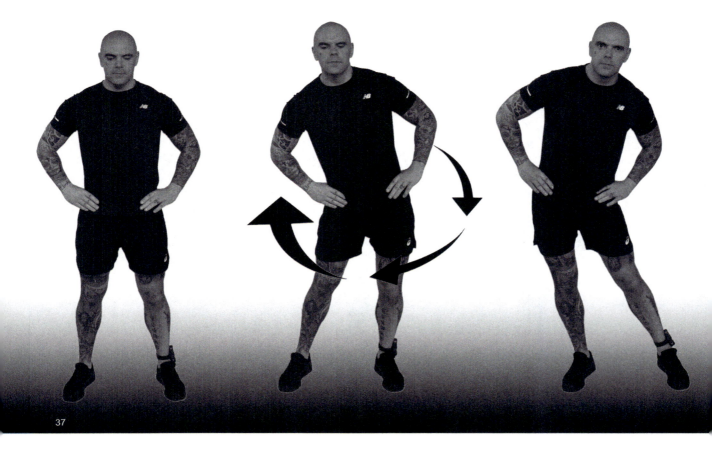

LEG SWINGS

Step 1: Standing upright lift one of your legs of the floor.

Step 2: Hold your arms out to keep your balance and swing your leg forwards and backwards.

Step 3: Alternate with your other leg for up to 2 minutes with short rests every 10 seconds.

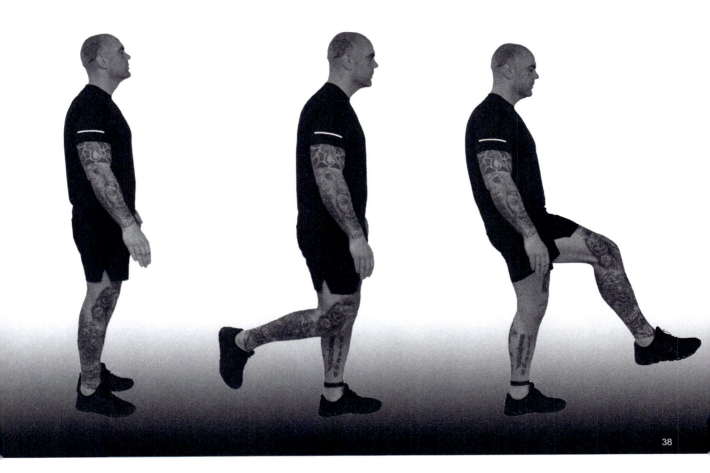

SPINAL ROTATIONS

Step 1: Stand with feet shoulder width apart.

Step 2: Lift your arms up in front of you to elbow height.

Step 3: Rotate your upper body to the left then to the right.

Step 4: Repeat a few times then rest then repeat again.

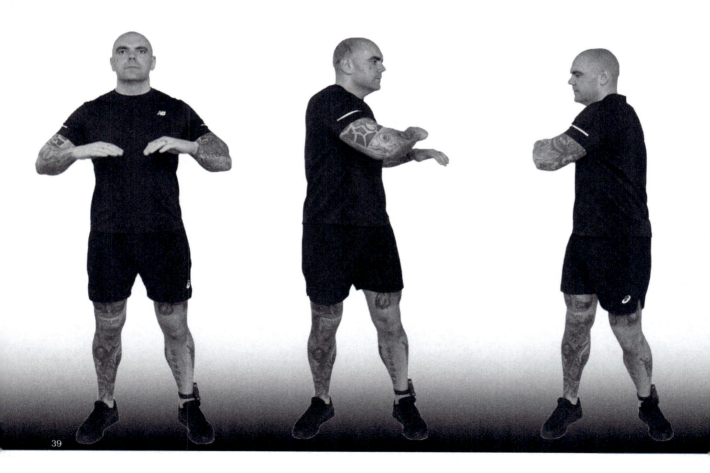

NECK CIRCLES

Step 1: Standing upright tuck your chin down towards your chest.

Step 2: Roll your head in a circular motion to loosen your neck muscles.

Step 3: Roll your neck the opposite way for up to 2 minutes with short rests every 10 seconds.

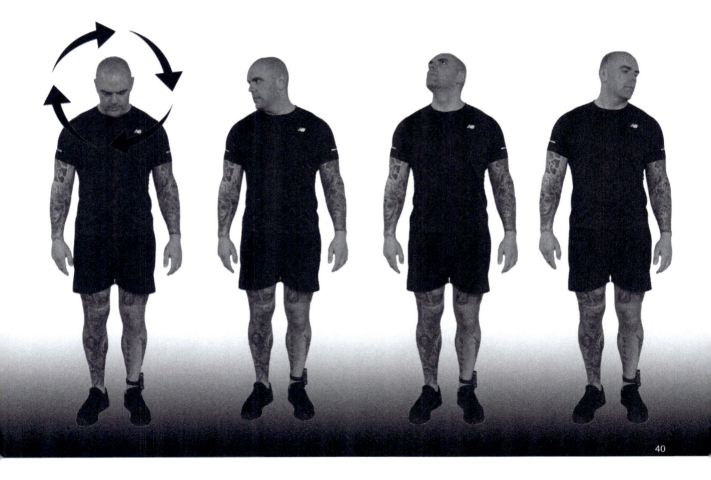

OVERHEAD TRICEP

Step 1: Standing upright lift your left arm up and place your hand behind your neck.

Step 2: With your right hand gently push your elbow and hold the stretch for up to 30 seconds.

Step 3: Repeat with your other arm.

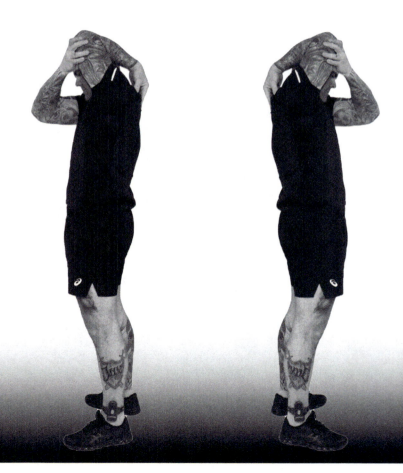

SHOULDER STRETCH

Step 1: Standing upright place your left arm across your body.

Step 2: Place your right forearm on your tricep and hold the stretch .

Step 3: Repeat with your other arm to stretch both shoulders.

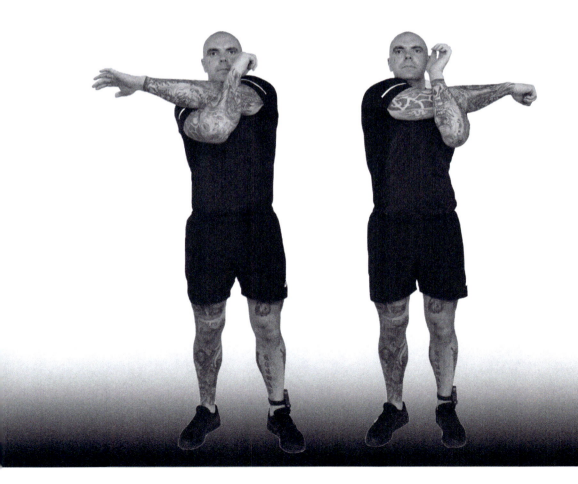

REVERSE SHOULDER

Step 1: Standing upright clasp your hands behind your back.

Step 2: Lean forwards slightly and push your arms up behind you gently.

Step 3: Hold the stretch out behind you for up to 30 seconds to stretch your shoulders and biceps.

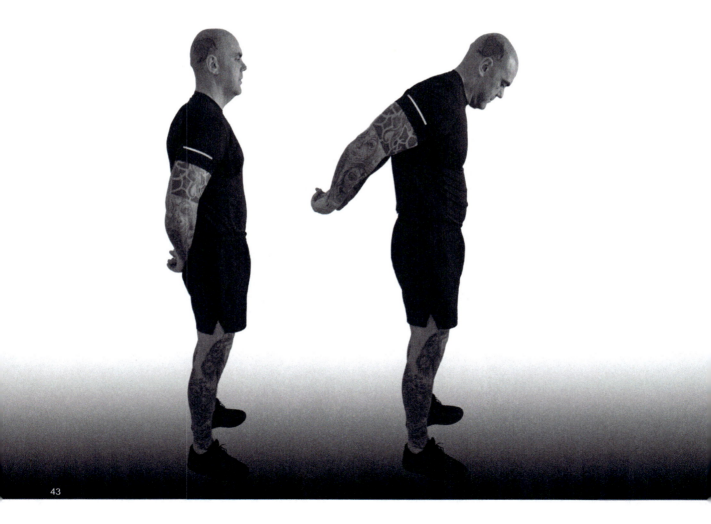

NECK FLEXION

Step 1: Standing upright tuck your chin into your chest.

Step 2: Hold the stretch for up to 30 seconds.

Step 3: Tilt your head backwards and hold the stretch for 30 seconds then rest.

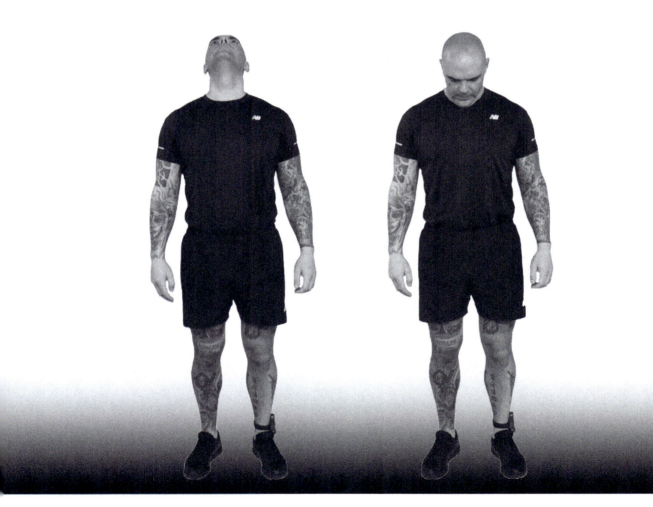

COBRA POSE

Step 1: Lie face down on the floor.

Step 2: Lift your head up and place your hands on the floor shoulder width apart.

Step 3: Tilt your head backwards and look up as you hold the stretch for up to 30 seconds to stretch your back, abs & chest muscles.

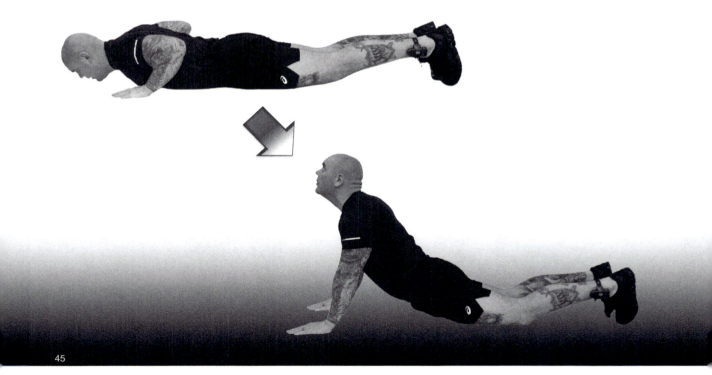

HAMSTRING STRETCH

Step 1: Lie on the floor on your back and lift your left leg up.

Step 2: Keep your leg straight and place your hands behind your calf and gently pull your leg towards you.

Step 3: Hold the stretch for up to 30 seconds.

Step 4: Repeat with other leg to stretch both hamstrings.

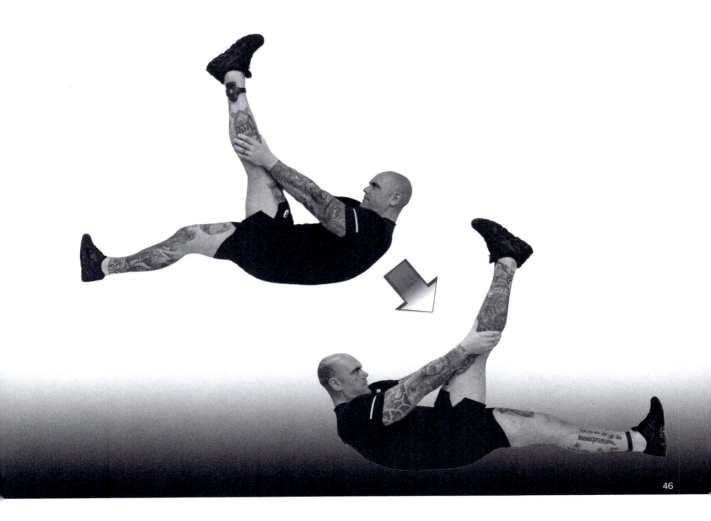

CALF STRETCH

Step 1: Standing upright place your left foot out in front of you.

Step 2: Point your toes up towards you and hold for up to 30 seconds.

Step 3: Repeat with other leg to stretch both calves.

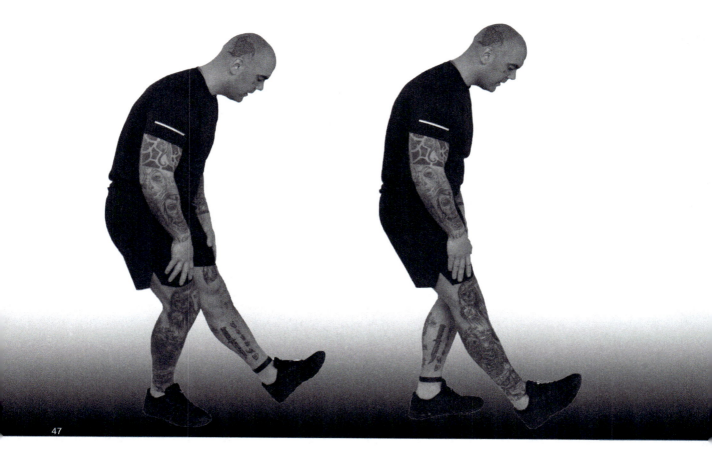

STANDING QUAD STRETCH

Step 1: Standing upright grab your left foot and pull it up behind you.

Step 2: Hold the stretch for up to 30 seconds and use your other arm for balance.

Step 3: Repeat with other leg to stretch both quads.

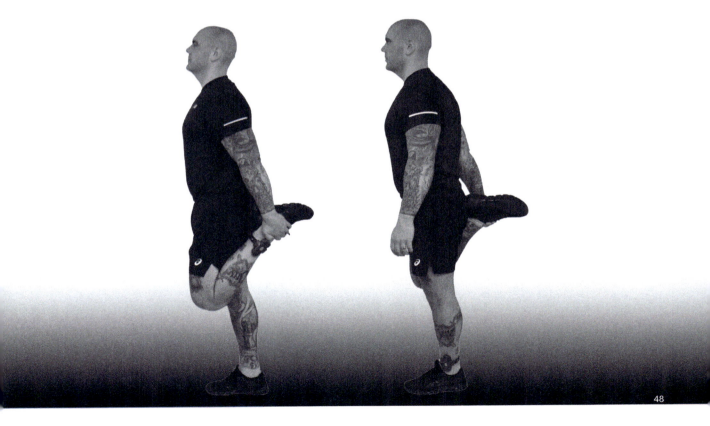

FORWARD BENDING

Step 1: Bend forwards gently trying to touch the floor.

Step 2: Hold the stretch for up to 30 seconds.

Step 3: Rest and repeat to stretch your back and hamstrings.

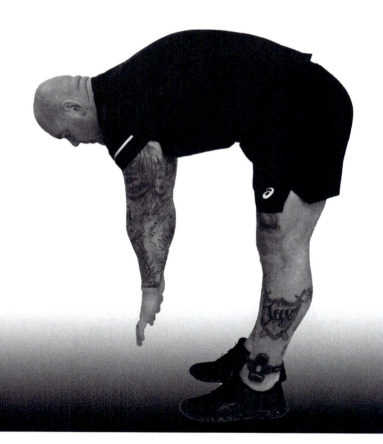

GROIN STRETCH

Step 1: Sit on the floor and place your feet together.

Step 2: Gently lower your knees out to the sides and push through your groin and press your feet together.

Step 3: Hold your feet and pull them towards your groin and hold for up to 30 seconds.

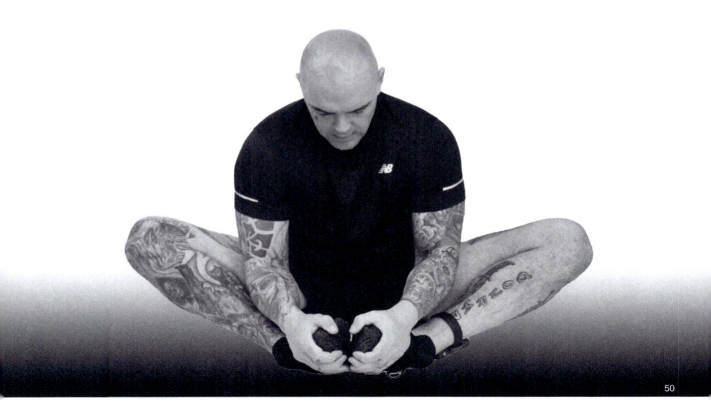

CAT & DOG STRETCH

Step 1: Get on all fours and create an arch in your back by raising your abdomen up and lowering your head.

Step 2: Hold the stretch for up to 30 seconds.

Step 3: Arch your back the opposite way by pushing your abs towards the floor and looking up to the sky.

Step 4: Hold the stretch for up to 30 seconds to stretch your back and spine.

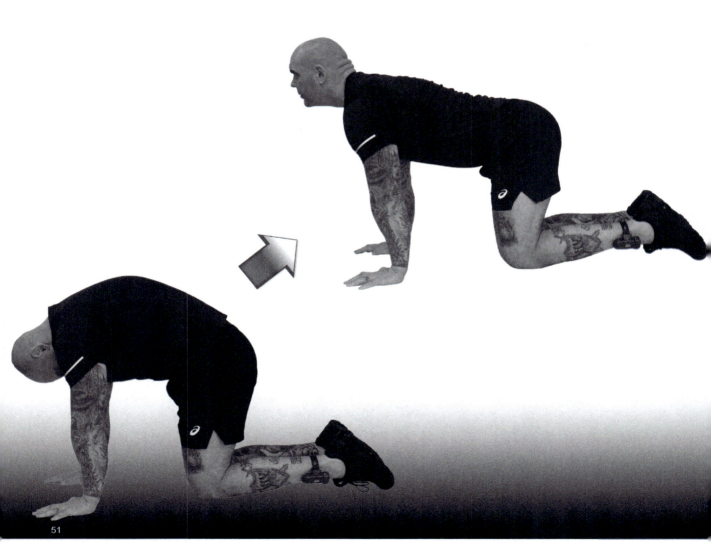

PEC & BICEP STRETCH

Step 1: Standing upright place your left hand on a wall palm down at shoulder height.

Step 2: Push your arm behind you and move your shoulder in towards the wall and hold the stretch for up to 30 seconds.

Step 3: Repeat with the other side to stretch both biceps and pecs.

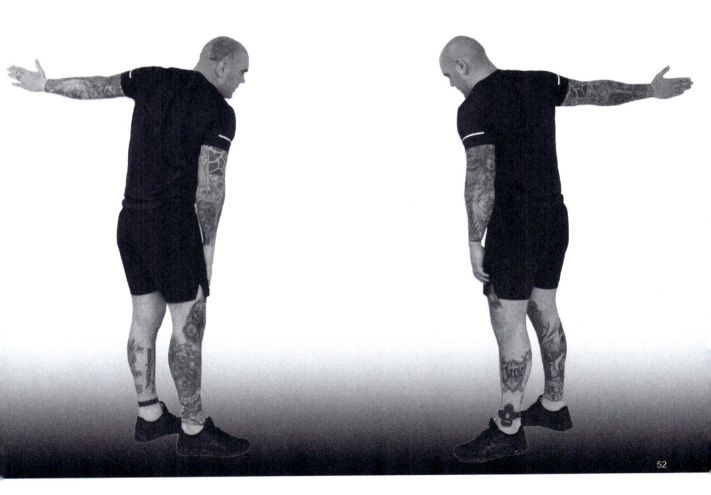

Walking, Jogging, Running & Sprinting

When most people think of fitness they think that it has to involve running but this is optional, but very beneficial. It is optional because you don't have to be a runner to be fit, as you can get fit from doing the workouts in this book.

Even walking on the yard for 30 to 45 minutes a day is so much
better for your health, fitness and again for your mental health. You won't believe how much better you feel by just going out for a walk, a good walk for 30 to 45 minutes and you soon start to clock the miles up.

If like a lot of people you don't like going on the yard at exercise time for whatever reason, it could be a mental health issue holding you back. It is just as beneficial doing it in your cell. You will be amazed at how much of a workout you can do by just jogging on the spot for 30 to 45 minutes. You can just zone out, forget about your thoughts and distract yourself from prison life as you do this.

You can increase the intensity of it as you get fitter by jogging on the spot faster and even doing interval training where you sprint for a minute, jog for a minute and repeat for 20 to 30 minutes. You will have such a sweat on by the time you finish you won't believe it. It's that simple to do a workout you just have to push yourself and have the determination and motivation to want to do it.

When you are jogging or running on the spot remember to be light on your feet, bring your knees up high in front of you and move your arms up and down fast as though you are out running on a track.

Next, I am going to list a few workouts you can try by just jogging on the spot and the benefits you will get from it are unreal. Even if you don't want to do the circuits just yet, you could maybe try this just to try and get your fitness boosted and your metabolism boosted to start burning through that excess fat from prolonged periods of bang up.

The benefits you will get from this is, first of all it will break your day up and get your heart working, pumping blood around your body and loosening them stiff joints up from sitting around. It will maybe ease the pain in your back from lying on them horrible mattresses all day. It will boost your mood and help get rid of them feelings of anxiety, stress, depression and help get rid of some of that pent-up anger and aggression as it focuses your thoughts towards working out.

Workout 1
Duration 30 minutes:
For the first 10 minutes just lightly jog on the spot. Speed up for the next 10 minutes. Then for the last 10 minutes lightly jog on the spot again.

- 10 minutes light jog
- 10 minutes fast jog
- 10 minutes light jog

Workout 2
Duration 45 minutes:
Lightly jog on the spot for 10 minutes.
Then for the next 30 minutes jog faster lifting your knees up higher.
Then lightly jog for the last five minutes.

- **10 minutes light jog**
- **30 minutes fast jog**
- **5 minutes light jog**

Workout 3
Duration 30 minutes:
This workout is a bit more intense and will really get you working and ridding them feelings of anxiety. This is an every minute, on the minute workout so at the start of every minute you will be sprinting on the spot for 30 seconds then jogging for 30 seconds, then sprint for 30 seconds, then rest for 30 seconds for a full 20 minutes.
This is ideal to do with your cellmate as you can take turns to sprint while the other is jogging.

- **5 minute light jog**
- **20 minutes (sprint 30 seconds, jog 30 seconds)**
- **5 minutes jog**

FITNESS TEST

To test your fitness and measure your progress do the following workouts, record your time and you will see how much progress you have made.

Do them on different days but they will really test your fitness, you will feel exhausted and will be gasping for breath after you have completed them.

The first is **100 burpees in as quick a time as possible**, do it at the start of your program and repeat it a month later and see how much you have progressed.

The next is **50 reps of each exercise:**

- **SQUATS**
- **SIT UPS**
- **BURPEES WITH PRESS UP AND JUMP**
- **LUNGES**
- **PRESS UPS**

Do it in that order and as quick as possible.

Another one is **100 press ups as quick as possible** to test your stamina and endurance, my best time on this was 1 minute 26 seconds.

You have to really push yourself on these fitness tests because they are brutal if you are giving it your all you will feel like giving up but with determination you will do it.

These tests will not only test your fitness ability it will test your mental strength as you will be gassing and feel like giving up. The beauty of these tests you can do them anywhere you want and doesn't have to be in the gym.

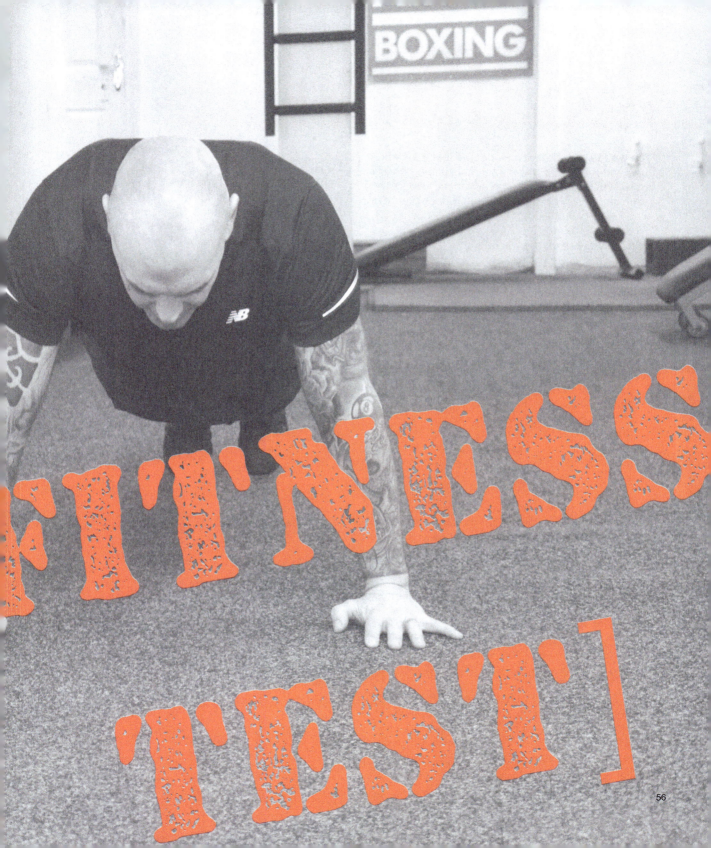

ABS TRAINING

When we talk about abs most people just think about sit ups and relate this to a 6 pack, this is the primary exercise but once you become advanced you will be doing exercises to target all 3 areas, upper abs, lower abs and side obliques.

The beginner ab workout will be for people just starting out as you need to strengthen your core before you can attempt to do the more harder exercises. I train my abs 3 times a week and this can be done in 20 minutes.

What I do is if I have time I will do them at the end of my circuit session or weights session as it doesn't use up too much energy. Don't get me wrong the workouts hurt and will leave you rolling around the floor but I don't class this as one of my workouts as it can be done within your workout or at the end of your workout. A lot of people think if you do sit ups your 6 pack will show up but it won't if its covered by layers of fat. It will strengthen your core and you will get a good set of abs but if you are overweight or have excess belly fat it won't show through.

Me personally I have never had a 6 pack that is protruding out as I've always been big and bulky, although I am trying my hardest now. I have a 6 pack and have an extremely strong core it just isn't sticking out but everyones different, some people are blessed with a 6 pack and don't even workout, sometimes it's all down to genetics but we can all do these exercises and strengthen and improve our core. All of the bodyweight exercises mentioned in this book have a role in strengthening your abs aswell because your abs come into play with every exercise you do so will be getting stronger with every circuit you do.

Sit ups target all of your abs but mainly your upper abs. Ab exercises where your using your upper body target your upper abs, ab exercises where you use your legs target your lower abs and exercises where you are turning or using your arms target your side abs (obliques).

Beginner Abs

Beginner abs will be targeting all 3 areas and will be 3 different exercises, it will be 3 sets per exercise and 10 reps if you can manage 10, if not just do as close to 10 as possible and build up to 10 every time you do them. So it will be a total of 9 rounds. You can add more rounds and reps once you can do this workout easy.

- **Sit ups 10 reps x 3 sets**
-
- **Leg raises 10 reps x 3 sets**
-
- **Heel taps 10 reps x 3 set**s

Six Hundred Abs

This is the workout I have in the 6 month fitness plan, it is 3 exercises and it is 10 sets per exercise with 20 reps. So do 10 sets of the first exercise before moving on to the next exercise.

- **Sit ups 20 reps x 10 sets**
-
- **Leg raises 20 reps x 10 sets**
-
- **Heel taps 20 reps x 10 sets**

Full Abs

All exercises are 20 reps each with a 1-minute Plank at the end of every round, rest for up to 2 minutes after every round, you will be doing 3 - 5 rounds depending on your ability. This targets the whole of your abs.

- Sit ups x 20
- Crunch twist x 20
- Bicycle crunch x 20
- Sitting twists x 20
- Leg raises X 20
- Full Plank x 1 minute

Lower Abs

This workout targets the lower abs and is 20 reps each exercise with a 20 second leg raised hold at the end of the round. Rest for up to 2 minutes at the end of the round. Do 3-5 rounds depending on your ability.

- Crunch kicks x 20
- Flutter kicks x 20
- Leg raises X 20
- Reverse crunch x 20
- Leg raised hold x 20 seconds

For time Abs

This workout is 1 minute each exercise for as many reps as you can do in a minute then rest for 30 seconds after every exercise. This will take you 15 minutes to complete.

- Sit ups
- Bicycle crunch
- Heel taps
- Leg raises
- Crunch twist
- Scissors
- Crunches
- Flutter kicks
- Sitting twists
- Mountain climbers

SITTING TWIST

Step 1: Sit on the floor with your feet out in front on you.

Step 2: Lean back slightly and embrace your core.

Step 3: Hold your hands together and try to touch the floor on your left side near your hip.

Step 4: Do the same on your right side and keep repeating from one side to the other, if your core is strong enough you can elevate your feet of the floor about a foot to make your abs work more.

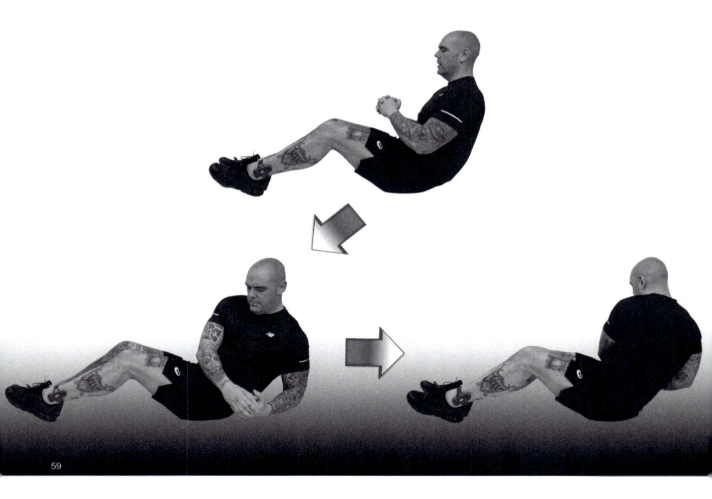

V SIT UPS

Step 1: Lie flat on your back on the floor.

Step 2: Crunch your abs together whilst reaching out with your arms fully extended.

Step 3: At the same time lift your legs of the floor and try to touch your toes so that your body is in a V position and your abs are crunching together.

Step 4: Lower yourself back to start position then repeat.

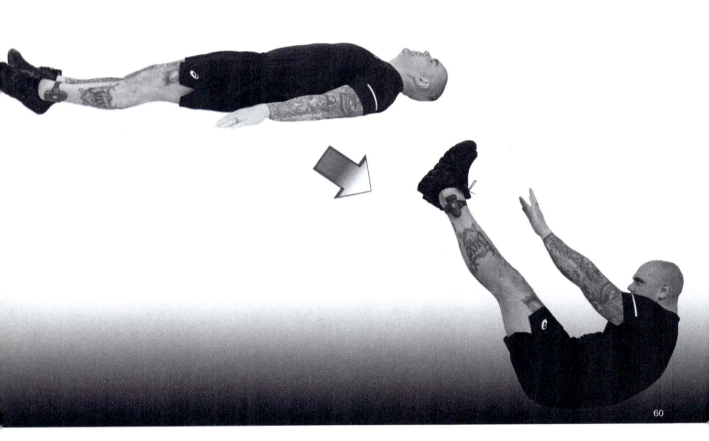

FLUTTER KICKS

Step 1: Lie on your back on the floor and lift your feet of the floor place your hands beside your hips palms down for stability.

Step 2: Kick your left leg about 2 foot higher then return.

Step 3: Then kick your right leg up and keep alternating doing flutter kicks whilst embracing your core.

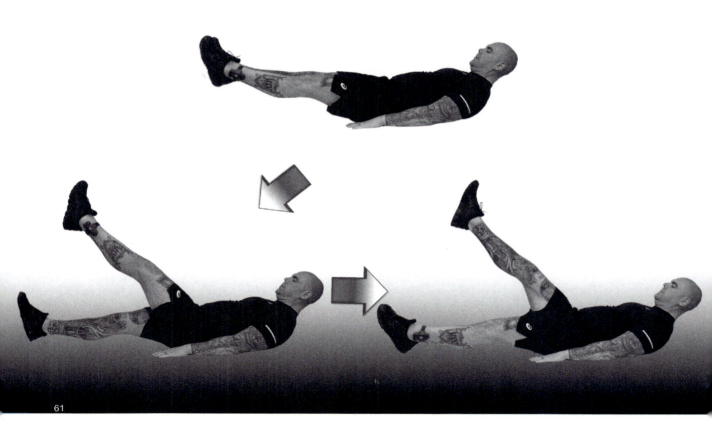

SCISSORS

Step 1: Lie on your back on the floor place your hands beside your hips palms down for stability.

Step 2: Raise your feet of the floor and spread your legs apart.

Step 3: Keep your legs straight and elevated and cross them over each other alternating legs over each other.

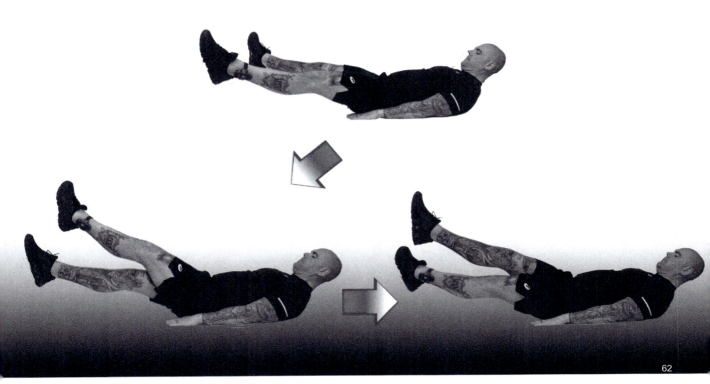

CRUNCH KICKS

Step 1: Lie on your back on the floor place your hands beside your hips palms down for stability.

Step 2: Crunch your knees up towards your shoulders.

Step 3: Kick your legs back out so that they are straight then repeat.

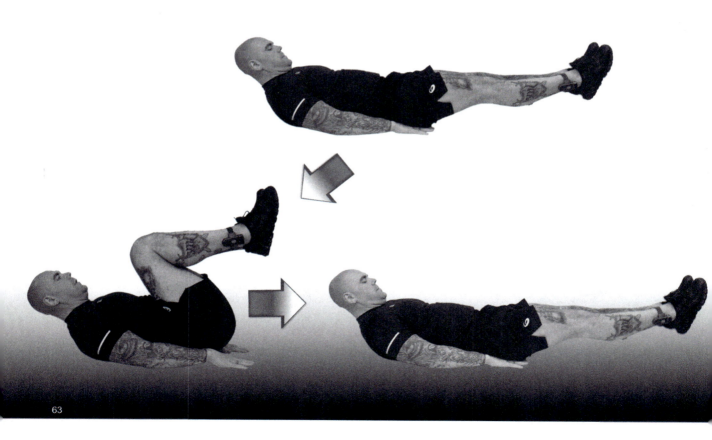

REVERSE CRUNCH

Step 1: Lie on your back on the floor, place your hands on the floor palms down and raise your legs in the air.

Step 2: Lift your hips of the floor, crunching your knees towards your head.

Step 3: Lower back to start position then repeat.

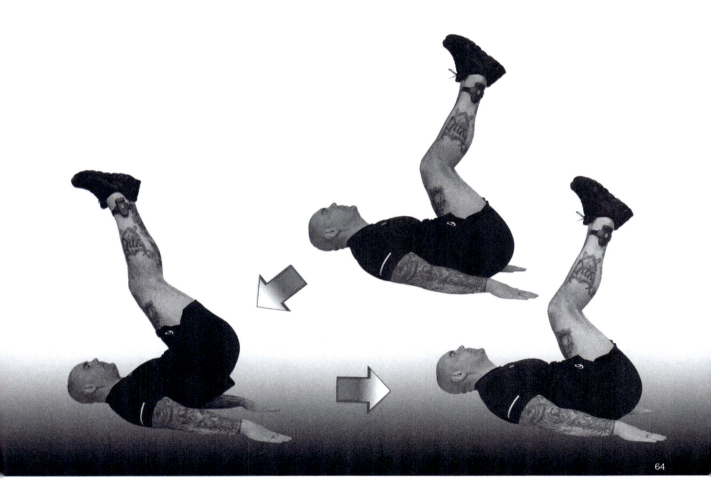

SIT UPS

Step 1: Lie on the floor on your back with your knees bent.

Step 2: Lift your shoulders off the floor and lift your upper body up towards your knees and touch the floor near your feet.

Step 3: Return to the lying down position. Then repeat.

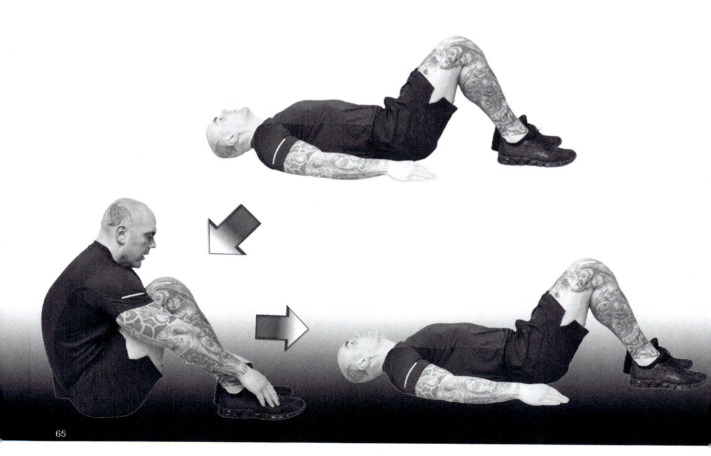

BICYCLE CRUNCH

Step 1: Lie on your back on the floor.

Step 2: Lift your feet off the floor so that you are in a crunch position.

Step 3: Begin pedalling as if you are riding a bike straightening your legs out as you do it. Then repeat.

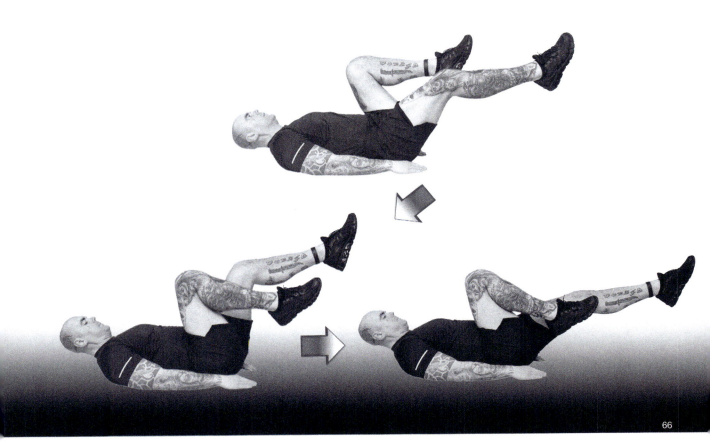

LEG RAISES

Step 1: Lie flat on your back on the floor.

Step 2: Put your hands at the bottom of your back for support and stability.

Step 3: Keep your feet together and lift them off the floor till your legs are at a 90° angle and return your legs back down but don't touch the ground, keeping the tension in. Then repeat.

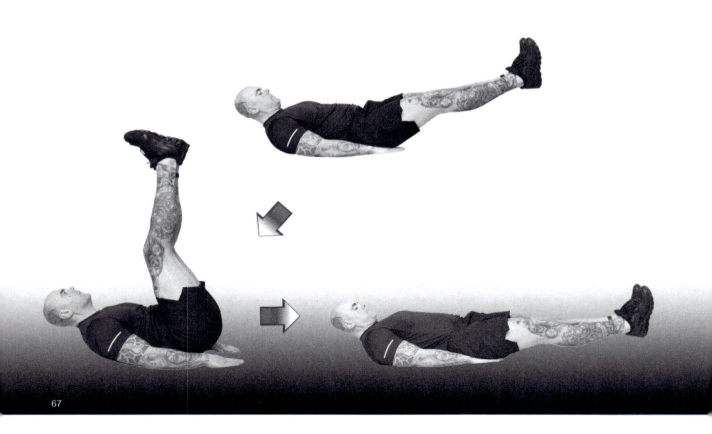

HEEL TAPS

Step 1: Lie with your back on the floor.

Step 2: Keep your knees bent and with one hand touch your heel.

Step 3: Repeat with the other hand touching the other heel. Then repeat.

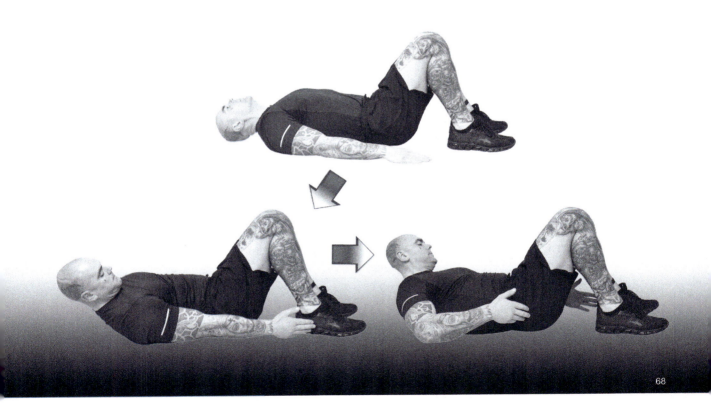

FULL PLANK

Step 1: Go down on your knees and put your hands on the floor shoulder width apart extending your arms out.

Step 2: Extend your legs out and engage your core and keep your body stiff.

Step 3: Hold this position for as long as possible.

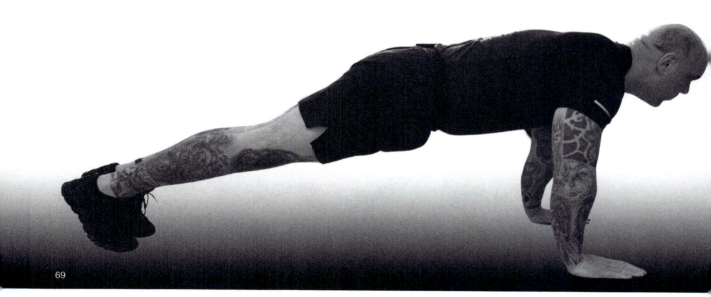

MOUNTAIN CLIMBERS

Step 1: Get in the press up position.

Step 2: Bring one knee up to your chest and return without touching the ground.

Step 3: Repeat with other leg. Then repeat.

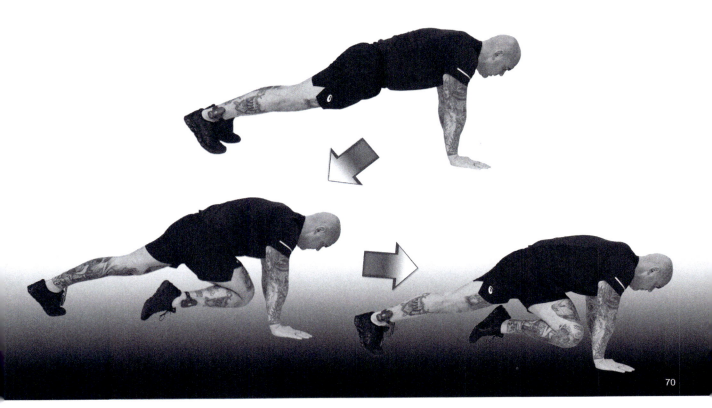

Cardiovascular Training

Low intensity long-duration: this is when you are working out at a relatively low intensity for a longer period where you are not getting out of breath, but you are training at a pace where you are still sweating, getting a good workout and feeling focused. This could be just jogging on the spot or on the yard at an easy pace for about 45 to 60 minutes.

Moderate intensity, medium duration: this is when you are working out harder but not giving it your all. This could be doing bodyweight exercises but not at your full capacity for around 30 to 45 minutes or running at a reasonable pace. This is designed to build up stamina and endurance.

High intensity, shorter duration: this is when you are giving it your all, going through a circuit as quick as possible in a shorter time or sprinting on the spot or on the yard. It could be a circuit that lasts 20-30 minutes or longer for the more advanced individual. In these workouts you will notice you are out of breath, sweating more and will feel aches. This is the lactic acid building up in the body which is normal for these types of workouts.

Anaerobic training: this is when you are training at maximum capacity for a matter of seconds and duration time is around 5 to 15 minutes. This is mainly sprinting which will be on the spot or on the exercise yard or treadmill. This could be sprinting for 20 seconds and resting 10 seconds then repeating the process until you are exhausted.

Weightlifting: this is when you are in the gymnasium using the weights to build muscle and improve your muscularity performance. It can be using either barbells or dumbbells, both are just as efficient as the other and sessions normally last about 45 minutes.

Yard equipment training: this is when you use the exercise frames that you have on the exercise yard, where you can do pull-ups, dips, sit ups and press ups which is really good way of training.

Circuit training: this is doing a number of different exercises one after the other for a set number of reps and repeating the process, adding a round every time. This is called doing a circuit. This can be done by using your own bodyweight or can be done in the gym with weights or a barbell with a set weight on the bar, which is then called weighted circuits or barbell circuit.

There are other types of training but these are the training types I will focus on in this book as I don't want to overload you with information and confuse you as a lot of books do.

I know from experience the types of training most of us like to do in prison is either bodybuilding, weightlifting, cardio, fitness training or sometimes a mixture of both. By following this book you can do what suits you best or even switch it up every few months so you don't get bored or used to the same exercise routines.

For those of you sitting in prison the majority of the time we are sitting or lying on our beds watching TV and gaining weight by the week. this is because you are not very active and eat a lot of rubbish food but without realising we can turn this around by doing exercises throughout the day. This will speed up your metabolism and enable the fat burning process as I know from experience when you come to prison your metabolism seems to slow down and you gain weight. This is more visible on your stomach, just look around, everyone seems to have the beer belly look, which is down to high sugary carbohydrate diet and inactivity.

By following these workout plans you will speed up your metabolism and begin to burn fat, feel more energised and less fatigued. It has been proven that by doing a high intensity workout you can continue to burn calories for up to nine hours afterwards.

Another great way of keeping yourself mobile throughout the day is by doing an exercise every time the adverts come on the TV throughout the day. For example do 25 press ups every time the adverts are on, that's 100 press ups in an hour. If you do that for five hours it adds up to a staggering 500 press ups throughout the day. It's easy enough to do it without using up too much energy and over a week that's 3500 press ups. WOW, what an achievement that is and you can easily do it if you put your mind to it, even if you can only do 10 press ups to start with, that amounts to 350 press ups over the week which is a good start.

So imagine setting yourself that goal and how good you will feel when you have achieved it and you tell your friends and family that this week you have completed 3500 press ups. The same goes for squats or any other exercise you want to do, it's all about setting yourself goals, sticking with them and accomplishing it. It's about being positive, determined and feeling in a better mindset.

PRISONER DUMBBELL WORKOUT

All you need for a prisoner dumbbell workout is 2 pillow cases and 8x 2 litre bottles of water or pop. 1 litre of water is 1 kilogram, so 8 bottles adds up to 16 kilograms in weight which is more than enough to do a dumbbell circuit or as I call them the prisoner dumbbells.

Maybe just start of with 2 bottles in each pillow case and as you get stronger add more bottles. You will be surprised because 4 bottles feels way heavier than an 8kg dumbbell but this is because of how the weight is spread out, whereas a dumbbell is just held either side of your hand the bottles are hanging down and the weight is moving as you lift it so it feels heavier.

Be sure to always have the bottles unopened and always take them out of the pillowcase when finished to avoid any conflict with the officers. A 2 litre bottle of pop from the canteen shop is only £1, therefore 8 bottles will be the best £8 you've ever spent.

These are the dumbbell circuits I do in my cell and you get an incredible workout done with them and you get an awesome pump on of them. The way I do these is supersets which is a combination of exercises together which adds up to a superset.

So I will do a superset have a minute or 2 rest then do another. I normally do 16 reps per exercise as you need to do more reps as the weight is light or you can do as many or as little as you feel comfortable with.

SHOULDER WORKOUT
Superset (10 rounds)
- Front raises x 16
- Side raises x 16

Then superset (10 rounds)
- Shrugs x 16
- Shoulder press x 16
- Upright rows x 16

ARM WORKOUT
Superset (10 rounds)
- Bicep curls x 16 (each arm)
- Behind neck triceps extension x 16

Then superset (10 rounds)
- Hammer curls x 16 (each arm)
- Triceps ski's x 16

LEGS
Superset (10 rounds)
- Dumbbell squats x 16
- Dumbbell lunges x 16
- Dumbbell calf raises x16

CHEST WORKOUT
Superset (10 rounds)
- Dumbbell press x 16
- Dumbbell flyes x 16
- Incline press ups x 16

BACK WORKOUT
Superset (10 rounds)
- Bent over rows x 16
- Upright rows x 16
- 1 arm rows x 16 (each arm)

FULL BODY WORKOUT
Superset (10 rounds)
- Dumbbell curls x 16
- Upright rows x 16
- Front raises x 16

Then superset (10 rounds)
- Behind neck tricep extension x 16
- Side raises x 16
- Bent over rows x 16
- Lunges x 16 (each leg)

SHOULDER + ARMS
Superset (10 rounds)
- Dumbbell curls x 16
- Front raises x 16
- Side raises x 16
- Upright rows x 16
- Tricep extension x 16

BACK + LEGS
Superset (10 rounds)
- Dumbbell squats x 16
- Bent over rows x 16
- Lunges x 16 (each leg)
- 1 arm rows x 16 (each leg)

Then superset (10 rounds)
- Upright rows x16
- Calf raises x16

Beginner Cell Workout

This is the beginner cell workout but can also be done in the gym, whichever you prefer. I will call it the beginner cell workout as this is what it is aimed at and can be done anytime of day with no equipment needed. For the experienced trainer this might seem easy but my aim is for someone who is brand-new to this and to break them in easy. It consists of 5 exercises with 5 repetitions per exercise which is a total of 25 reps per round. We are aiming for 5 rounds which is a total of 125 reps. This needs to be done 3 times per week on maybe Monday, Thursday and Saturday.

Do all the 5 exercises straight after each other and at the end of the round rest for a minute or 2 if need be then move onto the next round. This should be done in around 45 minutes and will be repeated for 3 weeks. The beginner cell workout lasts for 8 weeks by which time you will be capable of moving on to the more intense workouts. In weeks 4 and 5 you will add an extra round so will be doing 6 rounds in total but with only a minutes rest in between rounds.

Week 6 it will be 7 rounds, week 7 will be 8 rounds and week 8 will be 10 rounds. It may seem repetitive but persist with it and you will see the improvements week after week. By the time you get to week 8 you will be doing 500 reps for your full workout and you will be used to the exercises.

Weeks One - Three *(5 reps on every exercise, 5 rounds, 3 times a week)*
- BURPEES
- SIT UPS
- PRESS UPS
- SQUATS
- JUMPING JACKS

Weeks Four - Five *(6 reps on every exercise 6 rounds, 3 times a week)*
- BURPEES
- SIT UPS
- PRESS UPS
- SQUATS
- JUMPING JACKS

Week Six *(7 reps on every exercise 7 rounds, 3 times per week)*
- BURPEES
- SIT UPS
- PRESS UPS
- SQUATS
- JUMPING JACKS

Week Seven *(8 reps on every exercise 8 rounds, 3 times a week)*
- BURPEES
- SIT UPS
- PRESS UPS
- SQUATS
- JUMPING JACKS

Week Eight *(10 reps on every exercise 10 rounds, 3 times a week)*
- BURPEES
- SIT UPS
- PRESS UPS
- SQUATS
- JUMPING JACKS

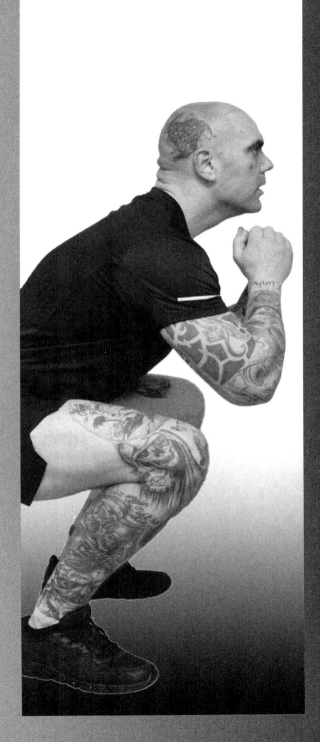

Yard Workout

The yard workouts can be done on the frames which we have on the exercise yard. You can do a back workout on the pull up bar with a range of different handgrips. These workouts can be done solely as your muscle group exercise if you don't go to the gym or as an extra session if you weightlift as well.

I always say to the lads if you can't or don't think you can do them start off with 2 pull-ups, the majority can do 2 pull ups if not get assistance and someone push you up, as you pull up. If you can only do 2 then do 2 then rest a couple of minutes and do another 2. Keep doing this until you can't do anymore, you might get three sets done, keep doing this a couple of times a week and after 2 to 3 weeks increase to 3 reps and repeat the process.

Before you know it after a couple of months you will be doing 10 reps. Same goes for dips on the dip bar, keep at it and you will progress. Progress is a long process but you will get there in the end. A good back workout will be 12 sets but the amounts of reps depends on the individual and can be lower reps for someone who is heavier.

Do four sets with an over hand wide grip. Four on the side grip and four sets on the underhand grip. I usually do reps of 10 reps as I am 110kg (17 stone), so that is a good rep range for me. Same for dips but do 10 sets of 10 reps, that is a good workout for your triceps and lower chest. Those are the two main workouts you can do on the yard with the frames. Me personally I like doing circuits on the yard as you can do laps of the yard as part of the circuit. It's so much better training in the fresh air when you are training hard and sweating.

This next workout which is done on the yard is an extremely good all round body circuit which works every muscle group and your muscles will be left aching after it. I have wrote it the way that I do it but you can change the number of reps you do for each exercise to suit you if you can't do that number of reps, but on the dip and pull up try to aim for 10 reps each round.

YARD BAR CIRCUIT ONE *(10 REPS X 10 ROUNDS)*
- **DIPS**
- **PULL UPS**
- **INCLINE PRESS UPS**
- **SIT UPS**
- **LUNGES**

Try to do it continuous without much rest or if need be take a rest at the end of each round for 30 - 60 seconds, before moving onto the next round.

The next circuits are similar, some are a bit harder if you include burpees and laps of the yard but again if it's too hard at first just do a set number of rounds. I would advise 4 to 5 rounds, do that once or twice a week and add an extra round every week until you can complete 10 rounds. It takes about 40 minutes to complete 10 rounds.

YARD BAR CIRCUIT TWO *(10 REPS X 10 ROUNDS)*
- **BURPEES**
- **PULL UPS**
- **SIT UPS**
- **DIPS**
- **UNDERARM ROWS**
- **PRESS UPS**
- **2 LAPS OF YARD**

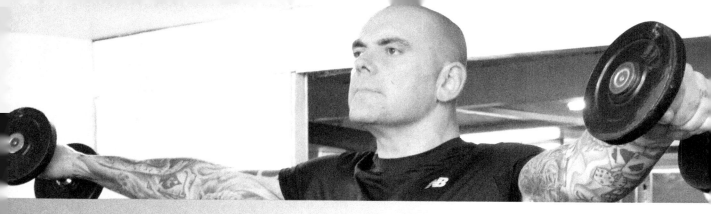

YARD BAR CIRCUIT THREE *(10 REPS X 10 ROUNDS)*
- PULL UPS
- DIPS
- PRESS UPS
- UNDERARM ROWS
- JUMP SQUATS *(deep)*

YARD BAR CIRCUIT FOUR *(10 REPS X 10 ROUNDS)*
- DIPS
- PULL UPS
- SIT UPS
- LEG RAISES
- PIKE PRESS UPS
- LUNGES
- 2 LAPS OF YARD *(or 200 meter run)*

If all of that seems too much for you or that isn't the workout for you because you feel you will lose too much weight and seems like too much cardio then this next workout is for you because it is less reps and not as many rounds. The exercises have to be performed more strict and slower so that you feel it more and will build more muscle.

YARD BAR CIRCUIT FIVE *(6-10 REPS X 5 ROUNDS)*
- PULL UPS
- DIPS
- UNDERARM ROWS
- PRESS UPS

YARD BAR CIRCUIT SIX *(10 REPS X 5 ROUNDS)*
- PULL UPS
- DIPS
- UNDERARM ROWS
- PRESS UPS
- SIT UPS
- SQUATS

Yard bar circuit 6 is the same as circuit 5 with 2 additional exercises. The reason for this is you have the choice whether you want to do sit ups and squats. It's better to do them but I know a lot won't want to do them, as your aim is to get bigger and you feel this will be too many exercises.

You can do 10 to 20 reps for press ups because the people doing this workout want to gain muscle, look bigger and doing more press ups gets you more pumped and makes you look bigger.

Working Out In The Gym

In this chapter I am going to talk about working out in the gym and lifting weights. I think for the majority of us, this is the preferred place to train as this is where we lift weights and ultimately get bigger.

First off, I'm just going to educate you on a vital fact. Your muscles don't get bigger in the gym they grow and get bigger when you are resting and eating the right foods afterwards. Most people think this happens inside the gym but when we are in the gym working out, we look bigger. This is what we call getting the pump on, when our muscles expand whilst training.

When we train in the gym our aim is to hit the five different muscle groups which is chest, back, arms, shoulders and legs. For beginners it is best to hit one muscle group at a time, that's one per session, sometimes we don't get enough sessions in prison to do this and have to hit maybe two muscle groups in one session.

This next workout plan is the basic exercises to target each muscle group. I am going to base it on four sessions as most prisons you get at least four sessions per week and this is purely weightlifting with no cardio for those wanting to gain extra muscle and increase bodyweight.

For the initial warm-up always do **20 reps** with just the bar or light dumbbells, then add some weight, do a second warm-up set and do 12 reps with this just to get the blood pumping and your muscles and joints warmed up.

Then you do **4 sets of 10 reps** on everything after that, you only need to do warm up sets at the start of each gym session.

On the bench press to start with just do **20 reps** with just the bar to get your chest and triceps warmed up.

On your second set pick a weight you can comfortably do **12 reps** with. These should be performed without a struggle and if you struggle the weight is too heavy.

For your next **4 sets** after this you should be pressing a weight where you can just get **10 reps**. If it's too hard then you need to take some weight off the bar. If it's too easy you need to add some weight to the bar. Same goes for the incline bench press, you should be getting **4 sets of 10 reps** with a decent weight that suits you.

The reason I am not saying a set weight amount is because we are all different, we will all have different starting weights and it's about picking the weight that best suits you to start with. When I first started on a bench press, I couldn't press 60kg and it took me well over a year to be able to bench press 100kg. You just have to train hard and your strength will increase. I will tell you later how to achieve this, this workout is a good starting point.

WARM UP SETS 20 REPS WITH BAR THEN ADD WEIGHT DO 12 REPS.

MUSCLE GROUP	EXERCISE	REPS	SETS
CHEST	BENCH PRESS	10	4
	INCLINE PRESS	10	4
	CABLE FLYES	10	4
TRICEPS	T-BAR PUSH DOWN	10	4
	ROPE PUSH DOWN	10	4

MUSCLE GROUP	EXERCISE	REPS	SETS
BACK	DEADLIFT	10	4
	FRONT LAT PULLDOWN	10	4
	REAR LAT PULLDOWN	10	4
	CLOSE GRIP PULLDOWN	10	4
BICEPS	HAMMER CURLS	10	4
	EZ BAR CURLS	10	4

MUSCLE GROUP	EXERCISE	REPS	SETS
SHOULDERS	SMITH MACHINE PRESS/ BARBELL PRESS	10	4
	DUMBBELL PRESS	10	4
	UPRIGHT ROWS	10	4
	FRONT RAISES	10	4
	SIDE RAISES	10	4

MUSCLE GROUP	EXERCISE	REPS	SETS
LEGS	SQUATS	10	4
	LEG PRESS	10	4
	LEG EXTENSION (ON MACHINE)	10	4
	HAMSTRING CURLS	10	4
	CALF RAISES	10-20	4

This is the weekly workout to target all muscle groups and they only need to be done once a week. A lot of us think the more we train one muscle group the bigger that muscle will get but muscles need time to grow and recover. After these workouts your muscles should be really sore to touch in the next few days afterwards. This is normal and just means you have trained properly. People say it doesn't happen after a while but believe me I've trained nearly 15 years and my muscles still ache like mad after a good workout.

If your muscles are not aching in the days after your workout then you haven't trained properly, it's as simple as that. So you should be doing this workout every week and all you have to change is the weight as you get stronger. After a couple of months you should be feeling stronger and the workouts will feel easier and this is when you increase the weight you are lifting. So if you were benching 40kg for four sets of 10 rounds you may want to increase it to 45kg or even 50kg if you feel strong enough.

These workouts are based on only getting to the gym four days a week but if you can get to the gym more days then do arms on a separate day and throw in some cardio as well.

After doing this workout for 3 months you will feel much stronger and will have gained some muscle mass. If your aim is to then bulk up more and get stronger you will want to move on to this next workout. In these workouts you will be lifting heavier weights with less reps and less sets. After your 2 warm up sets you will be doing 3 sets of 6 reps. If you can perform more than 6 reps then the weight needs to be increased and you should be doing 6 reps and resting for 2 to 3 minutes between each set giving you enough time to recover before doing the next set. For a lot in prison and I am talking from my own experiences, we want to get as big and as strong as possible. This is mainly the younger men. I have seen over the years that from the range of 18 to 30 most men (and I say men, as women don't you usually want to bulk up) want to get bigger and more muscular. The age 30+ want to get ripped and fitter. So what I will say about bulking up is that when you gain weight you want it to be good weight gain, muscle and not fat. The best way to do it is by eating good, healthy foods and plenty of good carbs like the foods I've mentioned in the nutrition section just more of it and over 3000 calories is a good start. The best sources of more carbs are oats, rice, pasta and fruit and veg. Don't get me wrong you can gain weight rapidly by eating the wrong foods but it is going to be excess fat. For instance if you eat loads of bread, chips, cake and custard you will gain weight quick but it will be fat storage. The best training for bulking is weightlifting and if you are new to weightlifting as long as you are lifting the weights properly and eating extra calories you are going to increase muscle mass and gain weight.

For bulking, the best training is doing lower reps with heavier weights, so I would suggest after your warm-up sets doing three sets of 6 to 8 reps with a weight that is heavy enough that you couldn't do 10 reps with. By doing this it will build muscle and strength plus aid in an increase in weight gain as you bulk.

It's also still important to do some cardio, even low intensity just to keep you mobile, heart healthy and to keep you fit, once or twice a week is sufficient. This can be a cell workout, doing a short circuit once or twice a week will not hinder your gains and will help you to keep in shape and be good for your mind and body.

Bulking Workout

MUSCLE GROUP	EXERCISE	REPS	SETS	REST
CHEST	BENCH PRESS	6	3	2-3 MINS
	INCLINE PRESS	6	3	2-3 MINS
	DUMBBELL FLYES	6	3	2-3 MINS
	CABLE FLYES	10	3	2-3 MINS
TRICEPS	CLOSE GRIP BENCH PRESS	6	3	2-3 MINS
	SKULL CRUSHES	6	3	2-3 MINS
	CABLE PUSH DOWN	10	3	2-3 MINS

MUSCLE GROUP	EXERCISE	REPS	SETS	REST
BACK	DEADLIFT	6	3	2-3 MINS
	LAT PULL DOWN	6	3	2-3 MINS
	CLOSE GRIP PULL DOWN	6	3	2-3 MINS
	BENT OVER ROWS	6	3	2-3 MINS
BICEPS	BARBELL CURLS	6	3	2-3 MINS
	DUMBBELL CURLS	10	3	2-3 MINS
	HAMMER CURLS	10	3	2-3 MINS

MUSCLE GROUP	EXERCISE	REPS	SETS	REST
SHOULDERS	SEATED SHOULDER PRESS	6	3	2-3 MINS
	UPRIGHT ROWS	6	3	2-3 MINS
	FRONT RAISES	10	3	2-3 MINS
	SIDE RAISES	10	3	2-3 MINS
	SHRUGS	10	3	2-3 MINS

MUSCLE GROUP	EXERCISE	REPS	SETS	REST
LEGS	SQUATS	6	3	2-3 MINS
	LEG PRESS	6	3	2-3 MINS
	LEG EXTENSIONS	10	3	2-3 MINS
	HAMSTRING CURLS	10	3	2-3 MINS
	CALF RAISES	10	4	2-3 MINS

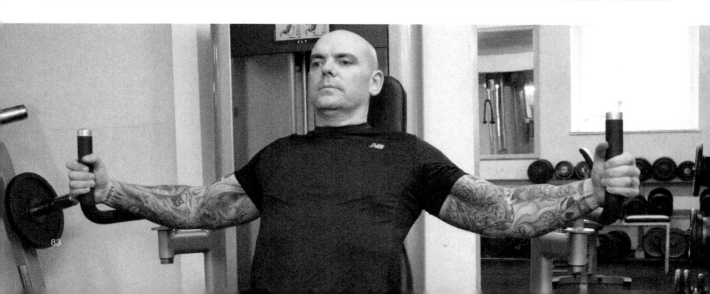

Cutting/Getting Lean

To become lean and shape up the best way, to do this is with a mixture of weights and cardio. This can be achieved alone by doing the cell workouts (circuits) but is best done with a mixture. Doing weights with a higher number of reps, and the rep range of 10 to 12, with four sets per exercise will help you tone up and get leaner. This can also be done by doing barbell circuits which will ultimately help you get fitter, stronger and leaner. You should be eating around 2500 to 3000 calories per day whichever suits you best, nothing is set in stone it's about trial and error and seeing what works best for you as an individual as we are all different. Try 2500 calories and if you feel like you want to stay the same weight you just want to get leaner try 3000 calories a day, because what works for me may not work for you. It's about getting the right amount for your body, but doing this type of training for a number of months will definitely get the desired effect. If your aim is to get lean and look more ripped you want to be doing more reps, more sets and performing more exercises with less rest in between sets. So after your warm up set you will be doing 4 sets of 12 reps. This will be done with a reasonable weight that you can manage 12 reps with without struggling. In between sets you will be resting for 1-2 minutes depending on the individual and how quick you can recover before performing the next set. After doing this workout your muscles will be really sore and will feel as though they have ripped. Your muscles are working more so eventually they will become harder and tighter giving you the lean and ripped look.

MUSCLE GROUP	EXERCISE	REPS	SETS	REST
CHEST	BENCH PRESS	12	4	1-2 MINS
	INCLINE BENCH PRESS	12	4	1-2 MINS
	DUMBBELL FLYES	12	4	1-2 MINS
	CABLE FLYES	12	4	1-2 MINS
TRICEPS	SKULL CRUSHERS	12	4	1-2 MINS
	T-BAR PUSH-DOWN	12	4	1-2 MINS
	ROPE PUSH-DOWN	12	4	1-2 MINS

MUSCLE GROUPS	EXERCISE	REPS	SETS	REST
BACK	DEADLIFT	12	4	1-2 MINS
	LAT PULLDOWN	12	4	1-2 MINS
	CLOSEGRIP PULLDOWN	12	4	1-2 MINS
	BEHIND NECK PULLDOWN	12	4	1-2 MINS
	BENT OVER ROWS	12	4	1-2 MINS
BICEPS	BARBELL CURLS	12	4	1-2 MINS
	EZ BAR CURLS	12	4	1-2 MINS
	DUMBBELL HAMMER CURLS	12	4	1-2 MINS

MUSCLE GROUP	EXERCISE	REPS	SETS	REST
SHOULDERS	OVERHEAD DUMBBELL PRESS	12	4	1-2 MINS
	BEHIND NECK PRESS	12	4	1-2 MINS
	UPRIGHT ROWS	12	4	1-2 MINS
	FRONT RAISES	12	4	1-2 MINS
	SIDE RAISES	12	4	1-2 MINS
	SHRUGS	12	4	1-2 MINS

MUSCLE GROUP	EXERCISE	REPS	SETS	REST
LEGS	SQUATS	12	4	1-2 MINS
	LEG PRESS	12	4	1-2 MINS
	LEG EXTENSION	12	4	1-2 MINS
	HAMSTRING CURLS	12	4	1-2 MINS
	DUMBBELL LUNGES	12	4	1-2 MINS
	CALF RAISES	12	4	1-2 MINS

One Rep Max

Doing your one rep maximum.

This is lifting your maximum amount of weight on any given exercise and is ideal to do when you first start training to see how much you can lift as well as maybe once a month just to see how much improvement you are making.

This must be performed after you are warmed up properly and with spotters, as it can be dangerous if you try to do it by yourself, so always have spotters. These are people that help you when you are performing the exercise, in case you can't lift it and it's too heavy. It's always good to test your strength to see how much you are improving and all of these workouts will ultimately help you gain strength.

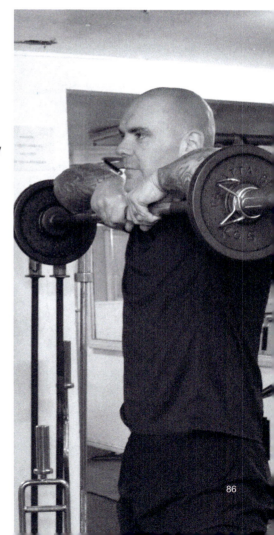

The SIX Month Weightlifting Cycle

This next chapter and workout routine is a 6 month routine and by the end of it you will be so much stronger and bigger. It starts off with higher reps and less weight but gradually the weights increase and the reps get lower. If you can do more reps on that week you are on the weight is not heavy enough and you need to increase it, as I said you are increasing the weight all the time as you are getting stronger when the weeks go on.

The compound exercises have less reps than the isolated exercises. The isolated exercises are the ones that hit the smaller muscles in the muscle group. The isolated movements are marked with a star* and they can be done with 10 reps. The compound movements hit the main muscle in the muscle group. This can be done in 3 months for an advanced individual but this is done over 6 month for beginners and people wanting to do a proper routine.

WEEKS 1 - 4: 4 sets x 12 reps

Weeks 5 - 8: 4 sets x 10 reps

Weeks 9 - 12: 4 sets x 8 reps

Weeks 13 - 16: 4 sets x 6 reps

Weeks 17 - 20: 3 sets x 4-6 reps

Weeks 21 - 23: 3 sets x 3-6 reps

Final week: you will be doing your max lifts. 1 rep max.

Below are the exercise you will be doing every week for this 6 month plan:

CHEST/TRICEPS
Bench press
Incline press
*DUMBBELL flyes**
*Peck deck**
*Cable flyes**
Close grip tricep press
*T-bar tricep extension**
*Rope tricep extension**

BACK/BICEPS
Deadlift
Lat pull down
Close grip pull down
Behind neck lat pull down
One arm rows
Barbell Curls
*EZ bar curls**
*Hammer curls**

SHOULDERS
Seated overhead press
Behind neck press
Upright rows
*Front raises**
*Side raises**
*Shrugs**

LEGS
Squats
Leg press
*Front leg raises**
*Hamstring curls**
*Calf raises**

By the end of this 6 month strength and power building cycle you will be much stronger, bigger and will be doing your one rep max at the end just to see how much strength you have gained.

Every 4 weeks you will be increasing the weight and lowering the reps to gain strength. The isolated movements don't have to be the same number of reps as you will already have done your strength training on the compound movements. The reps on the isolated movements can just stay at 10 but must also increase in weight as the weeks go on.

* Isolated Movements

The SIX Month Fitness Plan

WEEKS 1-4
The first 4 weeks will only consist of 4 Circuit sessions. This is to get you used to the exercises and to get used to the circuit routines and this is going to be the hardest part starting and continuing with it.

SESSION 1
THE FAST FIVE CIRCUIT.
You have to do as many rounds as you can in 30 minutes. You have to do at least 7 rounds so that you are pushing yourself. Do all 5 exercises 10 times through that is 1 round. Then repeat.

- BURPEES X 10
- SIT UPS X 10
- SQUATS X 10
- PRESS UPS X 10
- JUMPING JACKS X 10

SESSION 2
BURPEE SHUTTLES
You do 10 burpees followed by 4 shuttle runs which is 100m in length altogether. (So this can be done on the yard, in a car park, in the gym hall or if it's in your cell jog on the spot for 20 seconds). That's 1 round. Take a breather if needed then repeat. Do this for 30 to 45 minutes and add up your rounds. You want at least 10 rounds.

SESSION 3
THE FIVE HUNDRED CIRCUIT
The 500 circuit consists of 10 exercises with 10 reps and that is one round. We are doing 5 rounds of this which is 500 reps and will be doing this within 45 minutes.

- BURPEES X 10
- SQUATS X 10
- SIT UPS X 10
- PRESS UPS X 10
- JUMPING JACKS X 10
- CRUNCHES X 10
- TUCK JUMPS X 10
- SQUAT THRUSTS X 10
- STAR JUMPS X 10
- STEP UPS X 10

SESSION 4
THE DROP CIRCUIT
You can do this with a partner and do one person on one person off so you are resting when you are waiting for your partner to do their set. If it's by yourself have a 20 second rest after every set. You are doing 12 reps of each exercise then 10 then 8 then 5 reps and that is 1 round. You are doing 3 rounds in 45 minutes.

- BURPEES
- SQUATS
- PRESS UPS
- SQUAT THRUSTS
- TUCK JUMPS

12,10,8,5 reps x 3 rounds

So that is your first stage done and I have kept it relatively comfortable and you will be feeling fitter already after doing these workouts for 4 weeks. This is what these first 4 weeks will look like, you can pick what days you wish if you're doing them in the gym.

WEEKS ONE - FOUR

MONDAY - THE FAST FIVE CIRCUIT

WEDNESDAY - BURPEES SHUTTLES

THURSDAY - THE FIVE HUNDRED CIRCUIT

SATURDAY - THE DROP CIRCUIT

WEEKS FIVE - EIGHT

The next stage is weeks 5 to 8. This is when you will be stepping it up a gear and adding higher reps into the circuits and training 6 days a week. One of the days you will be doing a 5K run. This will be done on the yard, in your cell, in the gym on treadmill or out on the road. If you have to do it on the yard or in your cell it will have to be a jog on the spot if it's in your cell or around the yard for 30 minutes nonstop.

I do this myself, it is a good hard workout and will have you sweating. There will be 5 circuits with higher reps and the burpee shuttles will be the same, only you will be doing a minimum of 15 rounds and remember if it's in your cell or living room do a fast jog for 20 seconds after every set of burpees.

SESSION 1
THE FAST FIVE CIRCUIT

This time you will be doing more rounds and doing them faster and
with a minimum of 10 rounds or as many as you can in 30 minutes.

- BURPEES X 10
- SIT UPS X 10
- SQUATS X 10
- PRESS UPS X 10
- JUMPING JACKS X 10

SESSION 2
BURPEE SHUTTLES

Repeat these for 45 minutes and do at least 15 rounds. A lot of you will be doing more rounds maybe 20+ but 15 is your minimum goal.

SESSION 3
5K RUN

Or 30 minute run or run on the spot, whatever is available to you.

SESSION 4
THE SIX HUNDRED CIRCUIT

This is the same exercises as the 500 circuit with an extra 2 reps per exercise which is an extra 100 reps in total. 12 reps x 5 rounds.

- BURPEES X 12
- SQUATS X 12
- SIT UPS X 12
- PRESS UPS X 12
- JUMPING JACKS X 12
- CRUNCHES X 12
- TUCK JUMPS X 12
- SQUAT THRUSTS X 12
- STAR JUMPS X 12
- STEP UPS X 12

SESSION 5
THE DROP CIRCUIT TWO

This is the same exercises as the drop circuit, only the rep range has changed making it harder as you become fitter. Do 15 of each, then 12 of each, then 10 of each and then 5 of each. That's one round. Repeat 3 times.

- BURPEES
- SQUATS
- PRESS UPS
- SQUAT THRUSTS
- TUCK JUMPS

15, 12, 10, 5 reps x 3 rounds

SESSION 6
THE DOZEN CIRCUIT

This circuit is 12 exercises and will be 15 reps of each exercise, then 12 reps of each exercise then 10 reps, then 5. So you are going to do all 12 exercises 4 times.

- BURPEES
- SQUATS
- SQUAT THRUSTS
- PRESS UPS
- SIT UPS
- TUCK JUMPS
- STAR JUMPS
- CRUNCHES
- PIKE PRESS UPS
- DIPS
- HIGH KNEES
- STEP UPS

15, 12, 10, 5 reps

WEEKS FOUR - EIGHT

MONDAY - THE FAST FIVE *(minimum 10 rounds)*

TUESDAY - BURPEE SHUTTLES *(minimum 15 rounds)*

WEDNESDAY - 5K RUN

THURSDAY - THE SIX HUNDRED CIRCUIT

FRIDAY - THE DROP CIRCUIT TWO

SATURDAY - RECOVERY DAY

SUNDAY - THE DOZEN CIRCUIT

Now you have completed weeks 4-8 which is stage 2, you will now feel lighter, quicker and fitter then you have been.

You are now moving onto the stage when you add jumps and press ups to your burpee's and you will be doing more explosive moves like press up claps and crossfit burpee's.

You will now be training twice a day sometimes and you will have to do these exercises on the yard or if it's available in the gym. You will be doing pull-ups, dips, incline and decline press ups of a bench. Some of the circuits will be the same but again they will be higher reps to push yourself as you get fitter.

This is the stage when you will really see how much fitter and faster you are, it will still be hard but you will be ready for it. Remember it's never easy and it's all about that determination and mental strength.

SESSION 1
THE FIT FAST FIVE CIRCUIT
This is the same as the fast 5 circuit you have been doing, only this time you will be doing crossfit burpees. You will still be doing it in 30 minutes and as many rounds as fast as you can. You will be doing at least 12 rounds and you will be replacing sit ups with mountain climbers 10 each leg.

- CROSSFIT BURPEES X 10
- MOUNTAIN CLIMBERS X 10
- SQUATS X 10
- PRESS UPS X 10
- JUMPING JACKS X 10

SESSION 1 PART 2
PULL UPS
You will be doing 10 sets, 5 sets of wide grip pull ups and 5 sets of underarm pull ups with 10 reps if possible, if you can't do 10 then do whatever number of reps you are capable of doing but stay at that number for the full 10 sets and do this in 30 to 40 minutes.

SESSION 2
BURPEE JUMP SHUTTLES
This is the same as the burpee shuttles you have been doing, only this time you are doing them with a jump. You won't believe how much harder it is with a jump but you are now fit enough to be able to do these. This time you will still be aiming for at least 15 rounds. Remember if you need a rest do it after you have completed the shuttles.

SESSION 2 PART TWO
DIPS
This will be done in the afternoon when you have had a few hours in between the circuits so you are fresh. This can be done in your cell, house, prison yard, garden or in the gym. If it's in your house or a cell you can use two chairs or tables that are the same height and you will be doing dips 10 sets of 10 reps. You can take your time with these and get good form. You will get an unbelievable pump on your triceps and chest.

SESSION 3
5K RUN
(or 30 minute jog on spot)
This is the same as the previous week, only you will be timing yourself and beating your previous time. If it's on the yard do the same. If you can't time it or track your distance run faster for 30 minutes nonstop picking up your pace. If it's in your cell you will be pushing yourself harder than before.

SESSION 3 PART TWO
ABS
In this session you will be blasting your abs. To start, you will be doing 10 sets of 20 sit ups. Again this can be done anywhere. Next you will be doing 10 sets of 20 leg raises. Then you will be doing 10 sets of 20 heel taps. This will be done in about 45 minutes and you will really feel this on your abs.

- SIT UPS 10 sets of 20 reps
- LEG RAISES 10 sets of 20 reps
- HEEL TAPS 10 sets of 20 reps

SESSION 4
THE SIX HUNDRED PLUS CIRCUIT
This is the same as the 600 circuit, only this time you will be doing crossfit burpees and press up claps plus squat jumps. These additional variations will really make a difference and be much harder. This will take 45 to 60 minutes.

- CROSSFIT BURPEES X 12
- SIT UPS X 12
- SQUAT JUMPS X 12
- PRESS UP CLAPS X 12
- JUMPING JACKS X 12
- CRUNCHES X 12
- TUCK JUMPS X 12
- SQUAT JUMPS X 12
- STEP UPS X 12
- STAR JUMPS X 12

X 5 ROUNDS

SESSION 4 PART TWO
PRESS UPS

This will be done about 6 hours after your circuit, so you have time to recover. You will be doing these in sets of 5 for 20 reps in three different variations. You will do 5 sets of incline of a bench or chair, then you will do 5 sets decline of a bench and then 5 sets of 20 on the military press ups. This is a total of 300 reps and you will have an awesome pump on by the time you finish.

- **INCLINE PRESS UPS 5 X 20**
- **DECLINE PRESS UPS 5 X 20**
- **MILITARY PRESS UPS 5 X 20**

SESSION 5
THE BIG DROP CIRCUIT

This is the same as the drop circuit, only it will have higher reps per exercise and the burpees will be with a press up and you will be completing 3 rounds. It will take you up to 60 minutes to complete. Do 20 of each exercise then 15 of each exercise then 10 of each exercise then 5 of each exercise that's 1 round.

- **PRESS UP BURPEES**
- **SQUATS**
- **PRESS UPS**
- **SQUAT THRUSTS**
- **TUCK JUMPS**

20, 15, 10, 5
x3 ROUNDS

SESSION 5 PART TWO
STRENGTH MIX

In this session you will be doing five rounds of each exercise. To start with you will do 5 ×10 dips (bar dips) deep and slow with good form for chest and triceps. Then you will do 5 × 10 close grip pull up for back and biceps. Then you will do 5 × 20 press ups.

- **DIPS 5 X 10**
- **CLOSE GRIP PULL UPS 5 X 10**
- **PRESS UPS 5 X 20**

SESSION 6
THE DIRTY DOZEN

This is the same as the dozen circuit, only it starts with higher reps then the reps decrease but you do all the exercises 20 times, then 15 times, then 12 times, then 10 and that's the circuit complete. This time there is an extra set of crossfit burpees added in.

- **BURPEES**
- **SQUATS**
- **PRESS UPS**
- **SQUAT THRUSTS**
- **SIT UPS**
- **TUCK JUMPS**
- **CRUNCHES**
- **STAR JUMPS**
- **PIKE PRESS UPS**
- **DIPS**
- **CROSSFIT BURPEES**
- **STEP UPS**

20, 15, 12, 10

SESSION 6 PART 2
STRETCHING

In this session you will be doing the static strectches for at least 30 minutes and loosening up your muscles. Do the dynamic stretches to start of with for 15 minutes and then perform the 12 static stretches.

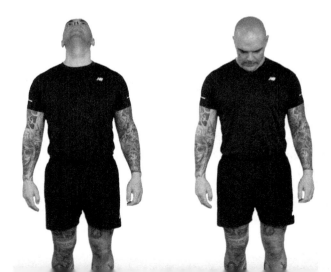

This is weeks 9-12 put together below what you have just read.

DAY	CIRCUIT SESSION ONE	SESSION TWO	WEEKS
MONDAY	FIT FAST 5	WIDE GRIP PULL UPS 10X10	9-12
TUESDAY	BURPEES JUMP SHUTTLES	DIPS 10X10	9-12
WEDNESDAY	5K RUN	AB WORKOUT	9-12
THURSDAY	600+	PRESS UPS 15X20	9-12
FRIDAY	THE DROP CIRCUIT	STRENGTH MIX	9-12
SATURDAY	RECOVERY DAY	RECOVERY DAY	9-12
SUNDAY	THE DIRTY DOZEN	STRETCHING	9-12

This is stage 3 complete, weeks 9 to 12.

By now you will be really fit, feeling like you need to peak and progress further in your fitness and in the next 12 weeks you will really flourish, you will feel like a real athlete which is what you are becoming and will be by the end of the 6 month plan.

At this point you might be feeling like you should be fitter than what you are but this is just part of the process. At some point in the following 12 weeks you will get to a point when you know and feel you are at your all time fittest you have ever been, you will feel awesome and you will love the workouts and they are now a part of your life.

You have to train to feel good about yourself because when you miss a day you will feel like you haven't achieved anything and make you feel like shit. Now that you are at that stage to progress further here is what you will be doing. Some of the circuits will be the same but harder and you will be doing the same circuits every week for 12 weeks. You will be that ultimate athlete at the end of this 12 week stage. In the first few weeks of this stage you will be trying to get more rounds and faster times so that you are improving every week. When you hit a personal best target you will be maintaining that target every session you do after that.

It doesn't matter that the circuits are the same week after week because you won't and can't get bored of them because they are just as hard every week. The monster circuit is a one I've added in for this stage because as the name suggests it is a monster circuit, takes me an hour to complete and is a really hard but really good circuit. 2 laps is equal to approximatley 150 metres and 8 shuttle runs back and forth across the yard is 200 metres.

MONSTER CIRCUIT

ROUND 1
- 2 laps running round yard (150 metre)

ROUND 2
- 2 Laps
- 10 press up claps

ROUND 3
- 2 Laps
- 10 press up claps
- 8 shuttles

ROUND 4
- 2 Laps
- 10 press up claps
- 8 shuttles
- 15 crossfit burpees

ROUND 5
- 2 laps
- 10 press up claps
- 8 shuttles
- 15 crossfit burpees
- 10 squat jumps

ROUND 6
- 2 laps
- 10 press up claps
- 8 shuttles
- 15 crossfit burpees
- 10 squat jumps
- 2 laps

ROUND 7
- 2 laps
- 10 press up claps
- 8 shuttles
- 15 crossfit burpees
- 10 squat jumps
- 2 laps
- 10 press up claps

ROUND 8
- 2 laps
- 10 press up claps
- 8 shuttles
- 15 crossfit burpees
- 10 squat jumps
- 2 laps
- 10 press up claps
- 8 shuttles

ROUND 9
- 2 laps
- 10 press up claps
- 8 shuttles
- 15 crossfit burpees
- 10 squat jumps
- 2 laps
- 10 press up claps
- 8 shuttles
- 15 crossfit burpees

ROUND 10
- 2 laps
- 10 press up claps
- 8 shuttles
- 15 crossfit burpees
- 10 squat jumps
- 2 laps
- 10 press up claps
- 8 shuttles
- 15 crossfit burpees
- 10 squat jumps

DAY	CIRCUIT SESSION ONE	SESSION TWO	WEEKS
MONDAY	FIT FAST 5 (minimum 15 rounds)	PULL UPS	13-24
TUESDAY	CROSSFIT BURPEE SHUTTLES (min 20 rounds)	DIPS	13-24
WEDNESDAY	5K RUN (fastest time)	PRESS UPS	13-24
THURSDAY	MONSTER CIRCUIT	AB WORKOUT	13-24
FRIDAY	THE BIG DROP (3-4 rounds)	STRENGTH MIX	13-24
SATURDAY	RECOVERY DAY	RECOVERY DAY	13-24
SUNDAY	THE DIRTY DOZEN	STRETCHING	13-24

Once you have completed the 6 month fitness plan it doesn't stop there, you will continue doing circuits, maintaining your fitness and you will always be improving. You can now do all the other circuits in this book and make up your own plan, as you will now have the knowledge on how to stay fit and how often you should be training. You will also now move on to the advanced circuits in the advanced circuits section as you will now have the fitness and capability of doing them and you will improve and test your fitness abilities.

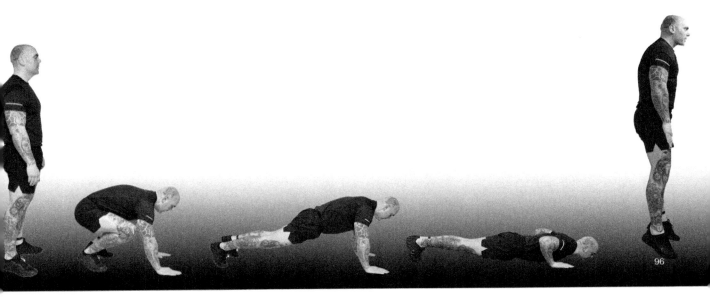

Additional Bodyweight Circuits

BODY ONE THOUSAND
20 reps all exercises 5 times through
- STAR JUMPS
- PRESS UPS
- DORSAL RAISE
- TUCK JUMPS
- STEP UPS
- BURPEES
- DIPS
- 180 BURPEES
- HEEL TAPS
- SQUATS

DECK OF CARDS CIRCUIT
Get a deck of cards and pick an exercise for each suit e.g
- HEARTS = BURPEES
- SPADES = PRESS UPS
- DIAMONDS = TUCK JUMPS
- CLUBS = SQUATS
- JACK = 12
- QUEEN = 13
- KING = 15
- ACE = 20
- JOKER = 80, 20 of each suit.

OVER FIFTY'S CIRCUIT

This is for the older people and less abled, do every exercise 10 times that's 1 round, rest for 2 minutes then do the same again, do 4 rounds. Thats 200 reps.
- JUMPING JACKS
- HIGH KNEES
- CRUNCHES
- HALF SQUATS
- PRESS UPS

TWENTY/TWENTY CIRCUIT

All exercises 20 times, 20 crunches after every exercise, followed by 1 minute Plank at the end of round. Do 3 rounds.
- STAR JUMPS/**CRUNCHES**
- PRESS UP/**CRUNCHES**
- CROSSFIT BURPEES/**CRUNCHES**
- JUMPING JACKS/**CRUNCHES**
- TUCK JUMPS/**CRUNCHES**
- SQUAT THRUSTS/**CRUNCHES**

FOR TIME WORKOUT

All 5 exercises is 1 round, complete 5 rounds and record your time, next time you do it you have to beat your previous time
- 50 JUMPING JACKS
- 40 SQUATS
- 30 SIT UPS
- 20 LUNGES
- 10 PRESS UPS

BURPEES, PRESS UP & SQUATS

- Do 5 crossfit burpees 10 press ups 15 squats X 20 rounds

Or you can do 10 crossfit burpees 20 press ups 30 squats X 10 rounds.
- Both ways add up to the same amount of reps.

THE PRISON NUTTER

- 50 STAR JUMPS
- 40 PRESS UPS
- 40 SQUAT THRUSTS
- 40 CRUNCHES
- 50 STAR JUMPS
- 40 PRESS UPS
- 40 SQUAT THRUSTS
- 40 CRUNCHES

REST FOR 1 MINUTE

- 50 STAR JUMPS
- 40 PRESS UPS
- 40 CROSSFIT BURPEES
- 40 CRUNCHES
- 50 STAR JUMPS
- 40 DIPS
- 40 ALT. SQUAT THRUSTS
- 40 CRUNCHES

ADVANCED CIRCUITS

These are the advanced circuits and you will only be able to do these and complete them once you are fit. You would not be able to do these unless you are already fit and are used to doing bodyweight circuits.

THE RUTHLESS BASTARD
- 10 BASTARDS – 20 PRESS UPS
- 10 BATSTATDS – 20 TUCK JUMPS
- 10 BASTARDS – 20 MOUNTAIN CLIMBERS
- 10 BASTARDS – 20 SIT UPS
- 10 BASTARDS – 20 JUMPING JACKS

Rest for 30 seconds after every 2 exercises, once you have
completed all exercises that's 1 round, do 3 rounds.

THE MEGA DROP
- CrossFit burpees
- Squats
- Press and clap
- Squat thrust
- Tuck jumps

25, 20, 15, 10, 5
Do all exercises 25 times each exercise then 20 then 15, 10 then 5, once complete thats 1 round do 3 rounds. Each round is 375 reps.

JUMP AROUND
Do all exercises 20 times then round 2 do 15 reps each
exercise then round 3 do 12 reps each then 10 reps for final round
- Press and clap
- Squat thrust
- Burpee's jump
- Star jumps
- Squat jumps
- Lunges
- Tuck jumps
- Squat thrusts
- Calf raises
- High knees
- Press and clap
- Burpee's jump
- Dips
- Bastards

20, 15, 12, 10

TEN OF THE BEST
- Squat jumps
- Sit ups
- Crossfit burpees
- Mountain climbers
- Tuck jumps
- Crunches
- Star jumps
- Lunges
- Leg raises
- Bastards

20, 15, 12, 10, 5

TWENTY TO ONE

- 20 x Burpees CrossFit
- 19 x Squat
- 18 x Press up
- 17 x Crunches
- 16 x Squat thrusts
- 15 x Burpees CrossFit
- 14 x Squat jump
- 13 x Press up
- 12 x Sit up
- 11 x Burpee's jump
- 10 x Squat thrust
- 9 x Star jump
- 8 x Crunches
- 7 x Press up
- 6 x Squat
- 5 x Tuck jump
- 4 x Sit up
- 3 x Press up and clap
- 2 x Burpee CrossFit
- 1 x Squat thrust

Go through all exercises one after the other, rest for a minute when you get to the bottom then go back up, rest for a minute then go back down, rest for a minute, then back up. 1 round = 210 reps 2 rounds = 420 reps 3 rounds = 630 reps 4 rounds = 840 reps.

BASTARD PARTNER

- 10 Bastards

Do this with a friend or in a group. Do 10 bastards then rest until your partner has done 10, that's 1 round. Do 30 rounds or go for time and keep going for 45 minutes.

SUPER SIX

- Crossfit burpees
- Alternate leg squat thrust x 10 each leg
- Star jumps
- Press and clap
- Tuck jumps
- V Sit ups

Do all exercises 10 times through, that's 1 round. Do as many rounds as possible in 30 minutes.

NAUGHTY FORTY

- Crossfit burpees
- Sit ups
- Tuck jumps
- Press ups
- Sqaut jumps
- Crunches
- Burpees
- Mountain climbers (20 each leg)
- Step ups
- Lunges (20 each leg)

Do all exercises 40 times that's 1 round. Do 2 rounds.

THE MULTIPLIER

You are adding another exercise every round with more reps

- 20 Crossfit burpees

- 40 Press ups
- 20 Crossfit burpees

- 60 Lunges
- 40 Press ups
- 20 Crossfit burpees

- 80 Sit ups
- 60 Lunges
- 40 Press ups
- 20 Crossfit burpees

- 100 Squats
- 80 Sit ups
- 60 Lunges
- 40 Press ups
- 20 Crossfit burpees

ADVANCED CARD CIRCUIT

- Hearts = Crossfit burpees
- Spades = Tuck jumps
- Diamonds = Press + clap
- Clubs = Squat jumps
- Jack = 12 reps
- Queen = 15 reps
- King = 20 reps
- Ace = 25 reps
- Joker = 80 reps (20 of each exercise)

This is what a deck of cards looks like which I turned over to make it easy for you if you want to copy it down and do yourself.

- 8 Clubs
- 6 diamonds
- 7 spades
- Jack spades
- 2 spades
- 6 hearts
- 6 spades
- 9 hearts
- 3 clubs
- King clubs
- Queen diamonds
- 2 hearts
- 4 diamonds
- 7 hearts
- Ace spades
- Queen clubs
- 7 diamonds
- 9 spades
- King spades
- Jack diamonds
- 8 spades
- 4 clubs
- JOKER
- 5 clubs
- 2 diamonds
- 9 diamonds
- 10 spades
- Ace spades
- 10 diamonds
- 3 hearts
- 4 hearts
- 3 diamonds
- 5 hearts
- Queen spades
- Queen hearts
- 10 hearts
- 6 spades
- King diamond
- 8 diamonds
- 4 spades
- King hearts
- 5 spades
- 2 clubs
- Jack clubs
- 5 diamonds
- Ace hearts
- 9 clubs
- JOKER
- 10 clubs
- 3 spades
- Jack hearts
- 8 hearts

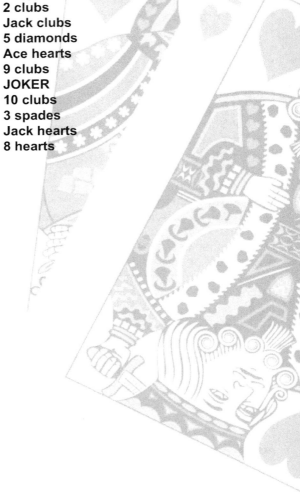

MY WORKOUT

The next workout program is what I was doing for 10 months from starting and I am still improving on my times and amounts of rounds I do. This is the way I have done it and I will explain to you how to improve and progress on it. I have mainly done the same workouts week in week out, but I have judged my fitness by the amount of rounds I added or the time I completed them in. Like I said everyone is different and some will advance quicker than others but we will all get fit by doing this workout. Most days I would train twice a day and I could do this by doing a circuit in my cell and when I was on the yard I would do a session on pull ups, sit-ups or dips.

	SESSION ONE	SESSION TWO
MONDAY	FIT FAST FIVE CIRCUIT	PULL UPS 10 X 10
TUESDAY	BURPEE SHUTTLES	DIPS 10 X 10
WEDNESDAY	MONSTER CIRCUIT	SIT UPS 20 X 10
THURSDAY	5K RUN	PRESS UPS 20 X 10
FRIDAY	THE DROP CIRCUIT	PULL UPS 10 X 10
SATURDAY	DAY OFF	DAY OFF
SUNDAY	DIRTY DOZEN CIRCUIT	DIPS 10 X 5 PULL UPS 10 X 5

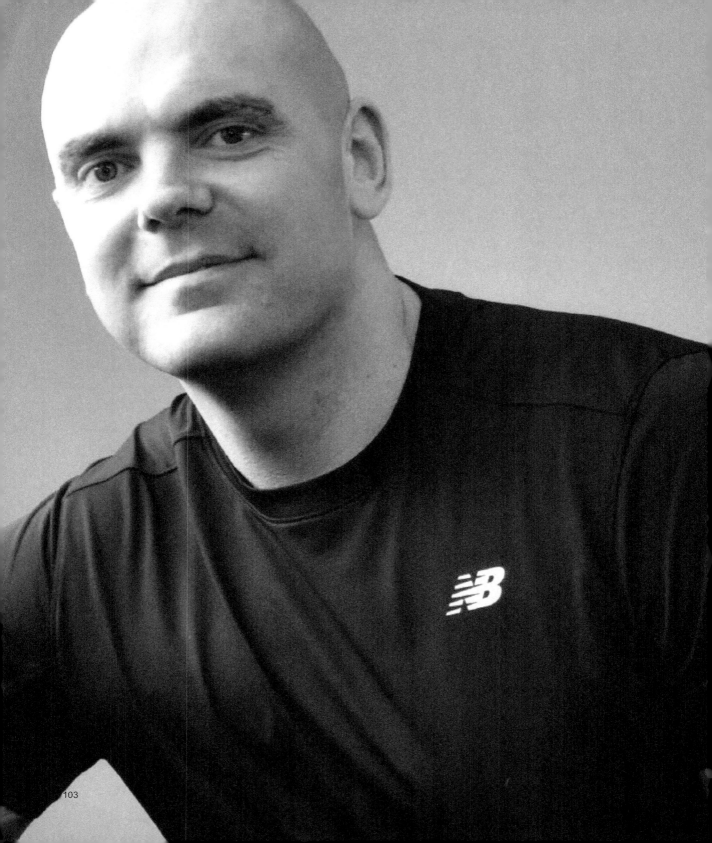

BARBELL CIRCUITS

This type of circuit training is done in the gym with a barbell and dumbbells and is a really good way of getting extremely fit and also building muscle.

Depending on your size and strength depends on what weight you will have on the bar but this is usually between 25kg and 50kg. Again it has different effects on your body as you do different weight and different amounts of reps. Usually if you do a 25kg circuit you will have a higher rep range and if you do a 50kg circuit the reps will be around 10 reps per exercise.

If your aim is to get bigger and fitter you will be doing the heavier circuits with less reps and if your aim is to be leaner, lighter and faster you will be doing less weight and more reps.

For the individual that wants to do these types of circuits you should start off with the lower weights and maybe still low reps but as you get fitter and stronger increase the weights and reps over the months so that you are always progressing.

The weighted circuit just like the bodyweight circuit are an all over body exercise and it targets every muscle in your body every session you do. This can be done with bodyweight circuits and other cardio as well but I would suggest doing at least four sessions per week along with a run and a bodyweight circuit for 6 months to see your full potential in this area. This is what a 6 month plan consists of.

THE SIX MONTH BARBELL CIRCUIT PLAN

All of the bodyweight exercises are 20 reps all the way through the 6 months and the weights are as follows:

Weeks 1-8 is done with 20-30kg for 20 reps.

Weeks 9-16 is done with 30-40kg for 15 reps.

Weeks 17-24 is done with 40-50kg for 10 reps.

DAY	CIRCUIT
MONDAY	POWER CIRCUIT
TUESDAY	ARM BLASTER CIRCUIT
WEDNESDAY	45 MINUTE RUN (at least 5k)
THURSDAY	BACK 2 LIFE CIRCUIT
FRIDAY	REST DAY
SATURDAY	SHOULDER BOULDER CIRCUIT
SUNDAY	BODYWEIGHT CIRCUIT (your choice)

POWER CIRCUIT

- POWER CLEAN AND PRESS
- STAR JUMPS
- BARBELL SQUATS
- PRESS + CLAP
- HIGH PULLS
- CROSSFIT BURPEES
- POWER CLEANS
- SQUAT JUMPS (bodyweight)
- SHOULDER PRESS
- LUNGES
- BENCH PRESS
- BASTARDS

X 3 ROUNDS

SHOULDER BOULDER

- POWER CLEAN + PRESS
- TUCK JUMPS
- DUMBBELL SHOULDER PRESS
- SIT UPS
- DUMBBELL SIDE RAISES
- CROSSFIT BURPEES
- DUMBBELL FRONT RAISES
- HIGH PULLS
- STAR JUMPS
- KETTLEBELL SWINGS (8-16kg)
- PIKE PRESS UPS
- CRUNCHES
- SQUATS (bodyweight)
- UPRIGHT ROWS

X 3 ROUNDS

ARM BLASTER

Use a set of dumbbells, weight varies with week, heavier dumbbells as weeks go on. 5-20kg.

- BARBELL CURLS
- BURPEES
- DIPS
- SQUATS (bodyweight)
- CLOSEGRIP BENCH PRESS
- DUMBBELL HAMMER CURLS
- SIT UPS
- SKULL CRUSHERS
- JUMPING JACKS
- POWER CLEAN + PRESS
- PRESS UPS
- CLOSEGRIP BARBELL CURLS
- DUMBBELL TRICEP SKI'S
- BURPEES
- CRUNCHES
- CLOSEGRIP PRESS UPS

X 3 ROUNDS

BACK 2 LIFE

- BENT OVER ROWS
- CROSSFIT BURPEES
- UPRIGHT ROWS
- SQUAT JUMPS
- PRESS UPS
- PULL UPS
- TUCK JUMPS
- DEADLIFTS
- SIT UPS
- ONE ARM ROWS (10 on each)
- LEG RAISES
- POWER CLEANS
- CRUNCHES
- BASTARDS

X 3 ROUNDS

ADDITIONAL BARBELL CIRCUITS

40KG SIX HUNDRED REPPER

10 reps each exercise X4 rounds
- CLEAN + PRESS
- FRONT SQUATS
- CURLS
- STAR JUMPS
- POWER CLEANS
- PRESS UPS
- PRESS BEHIND NECK
- UPRIGHT ROWS
- BURPEES
- SIT UPS
- PRESS FRONT + BACK
- SQUATS
- BENT OVER ROWS
- DEAD LIFT
- JUMPING JACKS

THE POWER CIRCUIT 25KG

20 reps each exercise X 3 rounds
- POWER CLEAN + PRESS
- STAR JUMPS
- BARBELL SQUATS
- PRESS + CLAP
- HIGH PULLS
- CROSSFIT BURPEES
- POWER CLEANS
- SQUAT JUMPS
- SHOULDER PRESS
- LUNGES
- BENCH PRESS
- BASTARDS

40KG CIRCUIT

15 reps each exercise X 4 rounds, step ups in between each exercise
- SHOULDER PRESS
- SQUATS
- STAR JUMPS
- UPRIGHT ROWS
- PRESS UPS
- CURLS
- BENT OVER ROWS
- POWER CLEANS
- BEHIND NECK PRESS
- CROSSFIT BURPEES

BODY AND WEIGHT

Weight varies, choose a weight that suits 40kg = 10 reps, 30kg = 15 reps, 25kg = 20 reps, whatever weight you choose do the full circuit at that weight and number of reps)
- STAR JUMPS – SHOULDER PRESS
- TUCK JUMPS-SQUATS
- PRESS UPS-UPRIGHT ROWS
- BURPEES JUMP-BENT OVER ROWS
- SQUAT THRUST-SHOULDER PRESS
- CRUNCHES-POWER CLEAN
- SQUAT JUMPS-CURLS
- BASTARDS-PRESS BEHIND NECK
- JUMPING JACKS-LUNGES
- SIT UPS-BENCH PRESS

THE ONE THOUSAND UP

Do 100 reps on each exercise alternating with partner after every 25 reps before moving onto next exercise, partner on bike or step ups, choose a weight that suits you.
- BENT OVER ROWS 25-25-25-25
- CURLS 25-25-25-25
- SQUATS 25-25-25-25
- STAR JUMPS 25-25-25-25
- SHOULDER PRESS 25-25-25-25
- POWER CLEANS 25-25-25-25
- CRUNCHES 25-25-25-25
- PRESS UPS 25-25-25-25
- UPRIGHT ROWS 25-25-25-25
- TUCK JUMPS 25-25-25-25

50KG STRENGTH CIRCUIT

10 reps each exercise X 3 rounds
- SQUATS
- SHOULDER PRESS
- CURLS
- BURPEES JUMP
- BENT OVER ROWS
- STAR JUMPS
- POWER CLEANS
- PRESS UPS
- UPRIGHT ROWS
- BEHIND NECK PRESS

20 BODY 15 WEIGHT

Pick a weight you can do 15 reps with and do 20 reps on the bodyweight exercise. Do 3-4 rounds, 10 step ups after every exercise.
- PRESS UPS
- SQUATS
- TUCK JUMPS
- SHOULDER PRESS
- BURPEES
- CLEAN + PRESS
- STAR JUMPS
- UPRIGHT ROWS
- SQUAT JUMPS
- BENT OVER ROWS

THE BAD BOY CIRCUIT 25KG

40 reps on all exercise
- CLEAN + PRESS
- CURLS
- SQUATS
- SHOULDER PRESS
- UPRIGHT ROWS
- BENT OVER ROWS
- TUCK JUMPS
- BURPEES
- CRUNCHES
- BEHIND NECK PRESS
- POWER CLEAN
- PRESS UP
- STAR JUMP
- FRONT SQUATS
- DORSALS
- SHOULDER PRESS
- BENCH PRESS
- TUCK JUMPS
- CURLS
- POWER CLEANS
- WIDE PRESS UPS
- SQUAT JUMPS
- ALT. SQUAT THRUSTS
- BENT OVER ROWS
- CLEAN + PRESS

HEAVY CIRCUIT INCREASE

Do all exercises 20 times with 25kg that's 1 round, then do all
exercises 15 times with 35kg that's round 2, then do all exercises 10 times with 40kg to finish round 3.

- CLEAN + PRESS
- UPRIGHT ROWS
- BASTARDS
- BENT OVER ROWS
- POWER CLEANS
- ALT. SQUAT THRUSTS
- SHOULDER PRESS
- SQUATS
- CURLS
- TUCK JUMPS

HEAVY BURNOUT CIRCUIT

Do all exercises 10 times with 50kg that's 1 round, then do all exercises 15 times with 40kg that's round 2, then do all exercises 20 times with 30kg to finish of round 3.

- SHOULDER PRESS
- SQUATS
- STAR JUMPS
- UPRIGHT ROWS
- BASTARDS
- BENT OVER ROWS
- CURLS
- PRESS UPS
- BEHIND NECK PRESS
- POWER CLEANS

FULL BODY BARBELL

Do all exercises 25 times, do this 4 times through, that's 500 reps. Do this with a weight that you find it difficult to do 25 reps with to make it hard.

- CLEAN +PRESS
- SQUATS
- CURLS
- BENCH PRESS
- DEADLIFT

DIRTY DOZEN WEIGHT

Do 12 reps on all 12 exercises that's 1 round, do 3 rounds, dumbbell step ups after every exercise.

- CLEAN + PRESS
- CURLS
- BENT OVER ROWS
- BURPEES
- SQUATS
- SHOULDER PRESS
- POWER CLEAN
- STAR JUMPS
- HIGH PULLS
- TUCK JUMPS
- UPRIGHT ROWS

THE 50KG KILLER

Do this with 50kg or a weight that you find it hard to perform 10 reps with, do 20 reps on the crossfit burpees and star jumps, do 3-5 rounds. Whichever you can handle.

- POWER CLEAN +PRESS
- CURLS
- SQUATS
- OVERHEAD PRESS
- CROSSFIT BURPEES
- DEADLIFT
- UPRIGHT ROWS
- BENCH PRESS
- STAR JUMPS
- CLOSEGRIP BENCH

BODYWEIGHT EXERCISES

Bodyweight exercises are the ideal way to get extremely fit without the need for any equipment. The beauty of these are that they can be done anywhere at anytime. These exercises combined, target every muscle in your body, so will leave you with the desired effect of toning your muscles and helps in producing a healthier mind & body.

I will now explain all the bodyweight exercises that I have done and will explain step by step for each of the exercises.

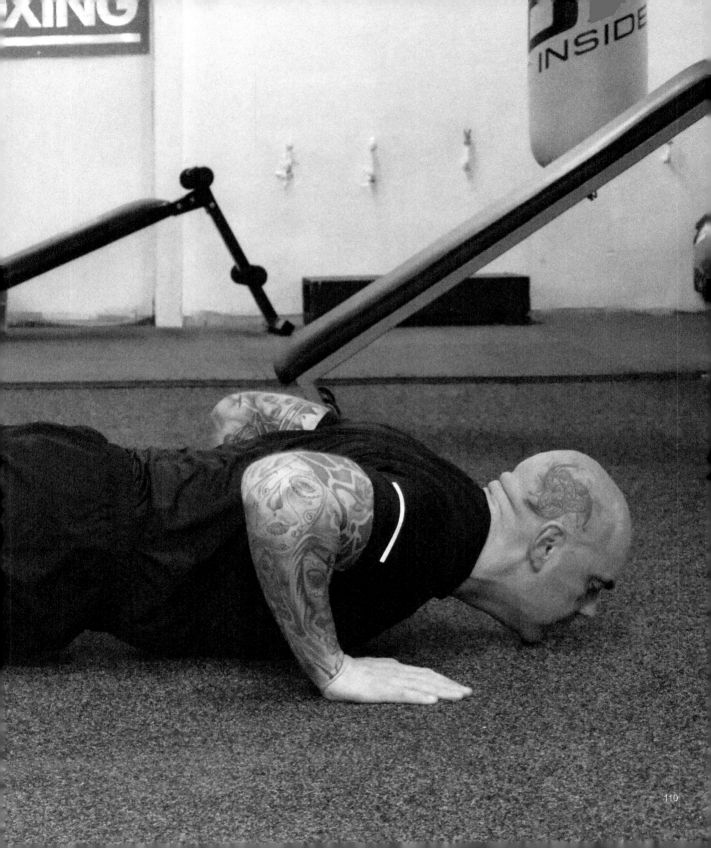

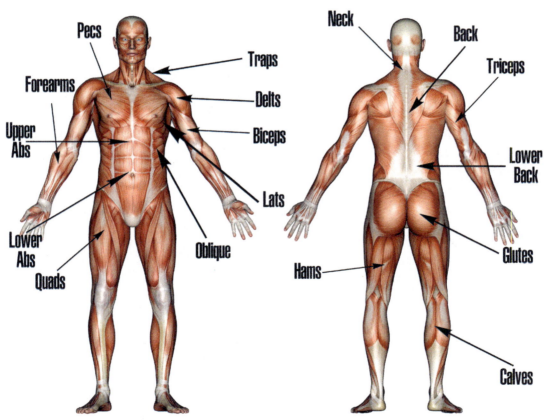

This image is showing the common names for all the major muscle groups. These are all the muscles you will be targeting in the following exercises.

BURPEES

This chapter is about burpees because burpees are the foundation of any fitness circuit and can be done in a variety of different forms.

Burpees are the primary exercise for circuits as they are the hardest exercise to do but also the best exercise to do. You either love them or hate them. People hate them because they are hard to do but once you master them you will love them.

I personally love them now but I will admit I used to hate them because they were so hard. So the different variations of the burpees are, first off is just a normal burpee. Then you have a **burpee jump**, where you do a jump at the end of a burpee. Then you have a **press up burpee**, where you do a burpee and press up in one go. The **cross fit burpee**, which is a burpee with a press up and a jump. The hardest of them all is a **Bastard**, perfect name for them as they are a bastard to perform. A bastard consists of a burpee into a squat thrust then press up then up into a tuck jump. This exercise is brutal and a circuit involving 10 to 20 of them in a round is enough to test the fittest of us all. Next we have the **180 Burpee** which is a burpee with a press up and 180 jump so you are facing the opposite way when you land on your feet. There are a few more variations of them but these are the most popular ones, the ones I will be using in my book and these are the ones which I use daily and you will be using.

To start off with you just do mostly the standard burpees which is more than enough for the beginner and when you advance and get fitter you move on to the more complex burpees. When I started doing bodyweight circuits like I mentioned before I detested the burpees but I changed my mindset towards them and dealt with them the way I deal with all my problems, head on. I started doing just burpees every day for about two weeks until I mastered them and felt comfortable with them. I made a circuit up called burpee shuttles, I'm sure it would of been around for years but on the yard I made a circuit where I would do burpees and then 4 shuttle runs per round.

Once you start to advance and you start enjoying burpees you can then add the press up or press up jump which is a crossfit burpee. When you do the crossfit burpees shuttle you will feel the difference but again, after you've been training for a few months then move on to this you should be aiming for about 15 rounds. This is the starting point for the advanced individual and try for 20+ rounds in 45 minutes.

Once you do these workouts you will love doing burpees. This is a very good workout and so simple to do for a whole body workout because the burpee targets every muscle in your body.

It targets the legs as you go into a squat, it then targets your chest and shoulder muscles as you go into the press up position. It is also targets your triceps and your abs as it engages your core helping you power through and up into a standing position. You will also feel it on your back and side lats as it engages every muscle in your body.

BURPEE

Step 1: Stand with feet hip width apart and squat down placing your hands on the floor shoulder width apart.

Step 2: Kick your legs out so you are in the press up position.

Step 3: Bring your knees back in towards your chest.

Step 4: Pushing through with your legs return back up into the starting position. Then repeat.

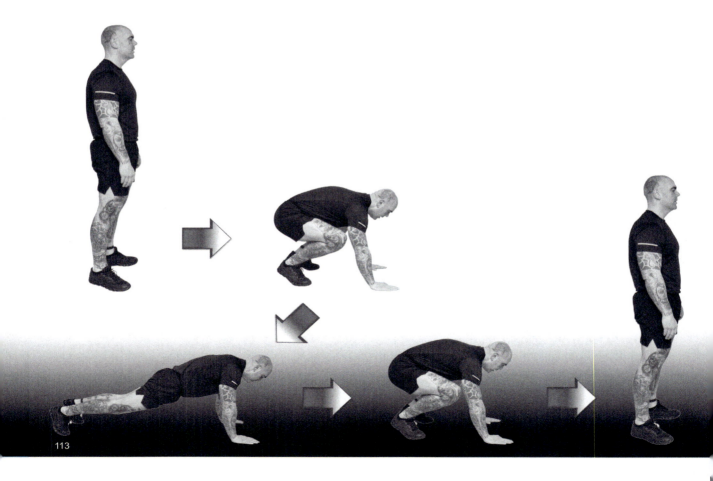

BURPEE JUMP

Step 1: Stand with your feet hip width apart and squat down placing your hands on the floor shoulder width apart.

Step 2: Kick your legs out so you are in the press up position.

Step 3: Bring your knees up back in towards your chest.

Step 4: Pushing through explosively as you come back up jump up so you lift off the floor and land lightly back on your feet. Then repeat.

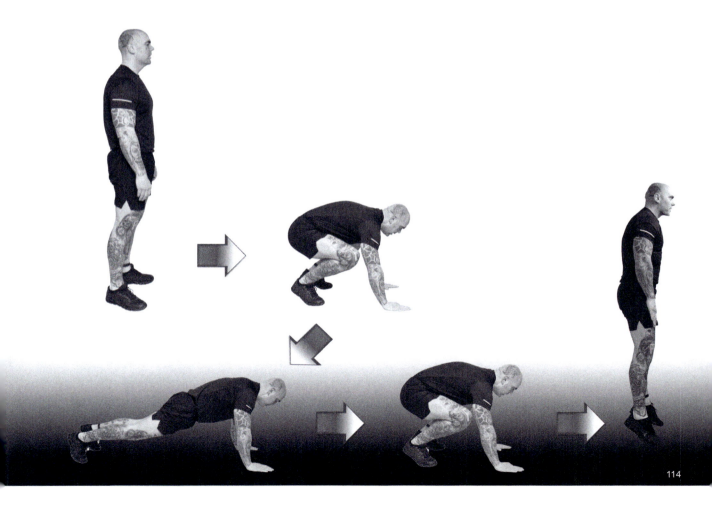

BURPEE PRESS UP

Step 1: Stand with your feet hip width apart and squat down placing your hands on the floor shoulder width apart.

Step 2: Kick your legs out so you're in a press up position then lower your body to the floor doing a press up.

Step 3: Bring your knees back towards your chest.

Step 4: Push through with your legs return back up into the standing position. Then repeat.

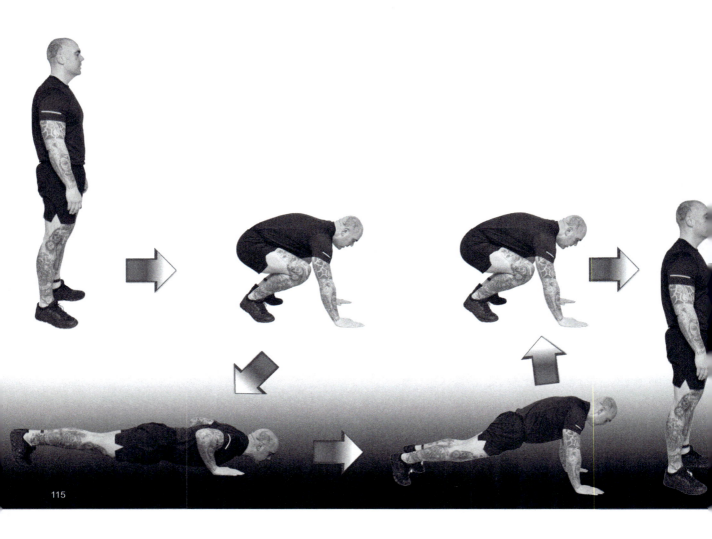

CROSSFIT BURPEES

Step 1: Stand with your feet hip width apart and squat down placing your hands on the floor shoulder width apart.

Step 2: Kick your legs out so you're in a press up position then lower your body to the floor doing a press up.

Step 3: Bring your knees back towards your chest.

Step 4: Push through explosively as you come back up and jump up so you lift off the floor and land lightly back on your feet. Then repeat.

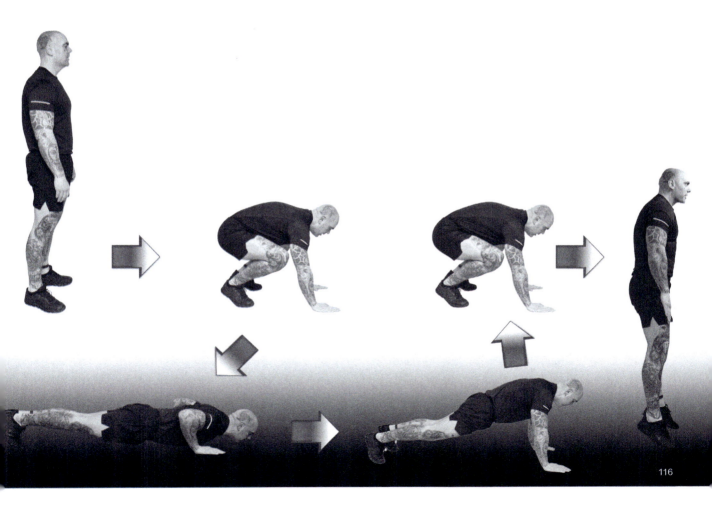

BASTARDS

Step 1: Standing with your feet hip width apart bend your knees and squat down placing your hands on the floor shoulder width apart.

Step 2: Kick your legs out so you are in the press up position.

Step 3: Bring your knees into your chest keeping your feet together placing your feet on the ground then kick your legs back out.

Step 4: Lower your body to the ground doing a press up and push back up.

Step 5: Bring your knees back up towards your chest and stand upright.

Step 6: Jump in the air bringing your knees up towards your chest tucking them in land lightly back on your feet. Then repeat.

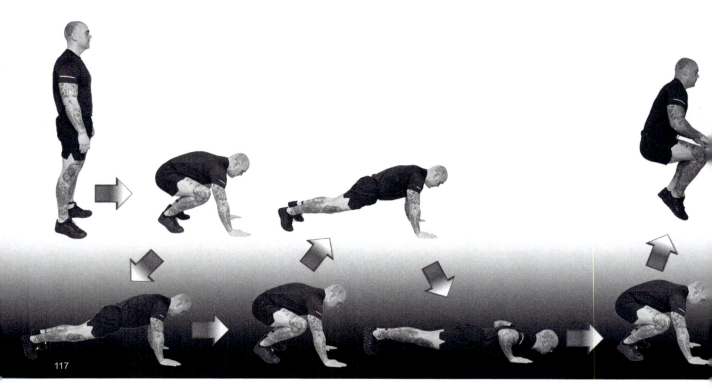

TUCK JUMP

Step 1: Standing upright facing forwards.

Step 2: Jump in the air bringing your knees up towards your chest tucking them in.

Step 3: Land lightly back on your feet and repeat.

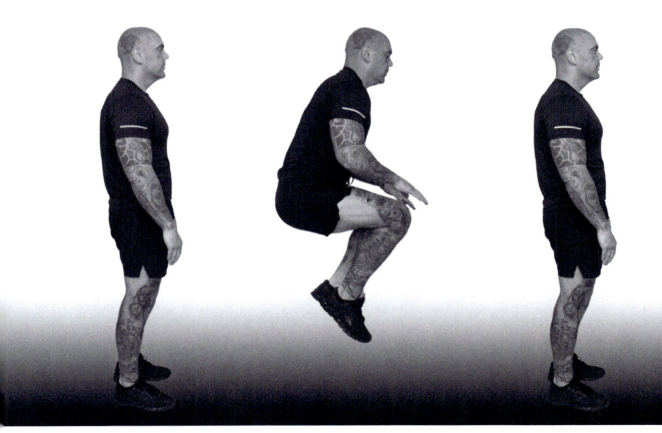

SQUAT

Step 1: Standing upright and facing forwards.

Step 2: Squat down so that your thighs are parallel with the floor. Holding your arms out in front of you to keep your balance.

Step 3: Keep your head facing forward and push back through your heels until you are standing upright facing forward.

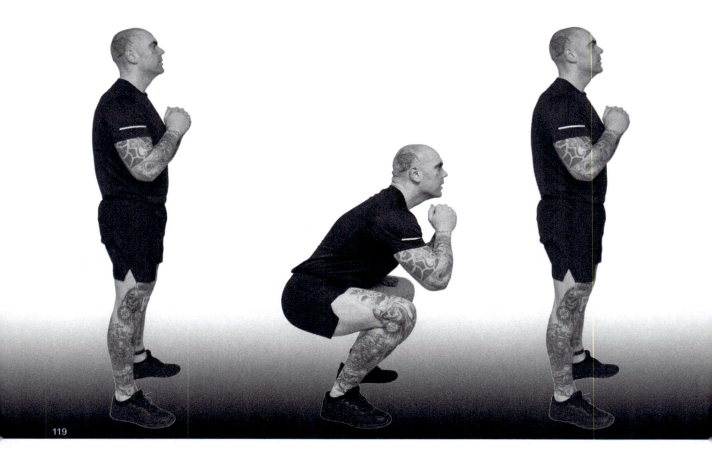

SQUAT THRUST

Step 1: Get in the press up position

Step 2: Bring your knees into your chest keeping your feet together placing feet on the ground.

Step 3: Kick your feet back out returning to the press up position. Then repeat.

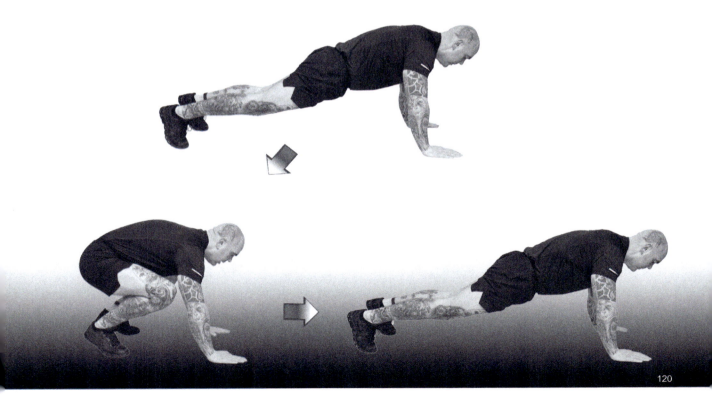

ALTERNATE LEG SQUAT THRUST

Step 1: Get in the press up position.

Step 2: Bring one knee up to your chest and place foot on the floor.

Step 3: Kick your foot back returning to the press up position. Repeat with other leg. Then repeat.

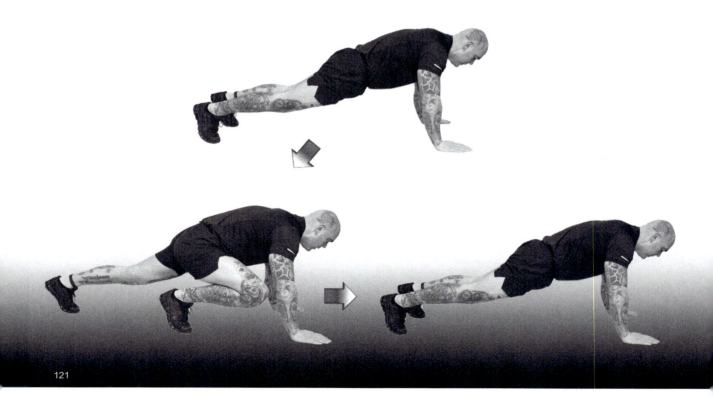

LUNGES

Step 1: Standing upright facing forward with feet hip width apart.

Step 2: Place one foot forward.

Step 3: Lower yourself with both knees bending your rear knee nearly touching the floor. Keep your arms out to the side to keep your balance

Step 4: Push up through your front leg returning to the standing position. Repeat with the other leg. Then repeat.

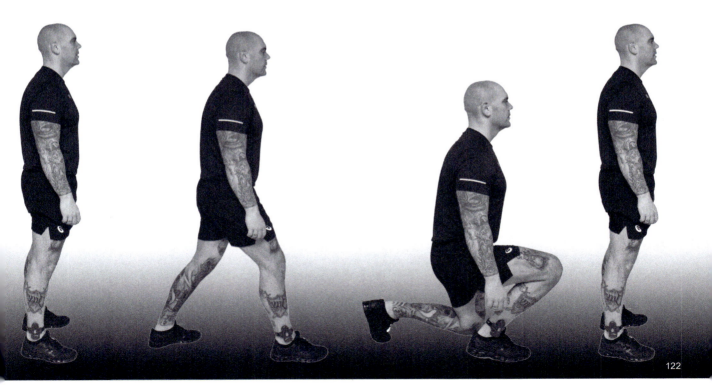

STAR JUMPS

Step 1: Standing with your feet together bend down with knees and touch the side of your shins.

Step 2: Push up through into an explosive jump, jump off the ground bringing your arms out to the side up to shoulder height and at the same time open your legs as you leave the ground.

Step 3: Land softly back on the ground. Then repeat.

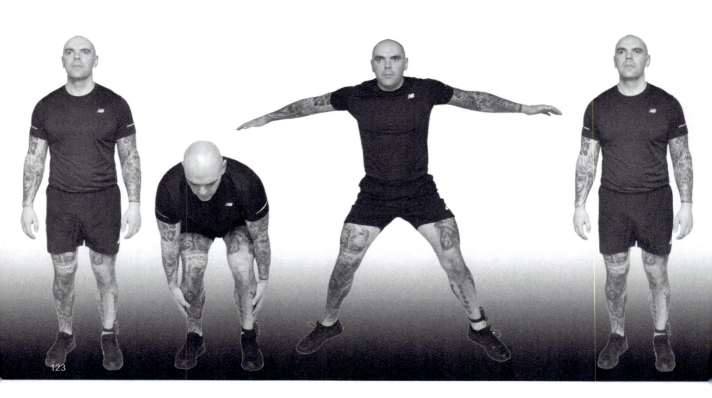

MOUNTAIN CLIMBERS

Step 1: Get in the press up position.

Step 2: Bring one knee up to your chest and return without touching the ground.

Step 3: Repeat with other leg. Then repeat.

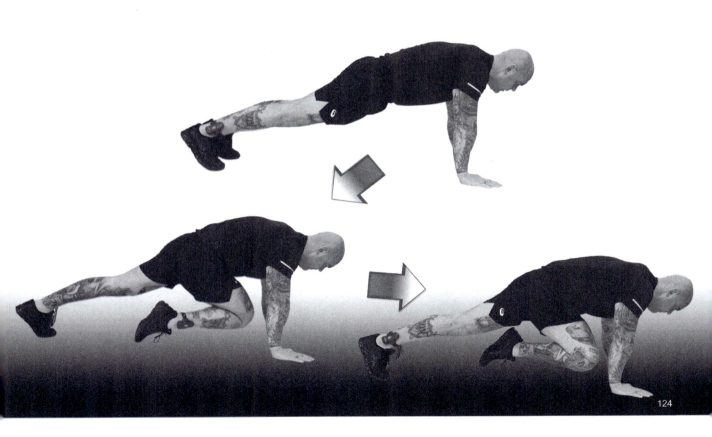

SIT UP

Step 1: Lie on the floor on your back with your knees bent.

Step 2: Lift your shoulders off the floor and lift your upper body up towards your knees and touch the floor near your feet.

Step 3: Return to the lying down position. Then repeat.

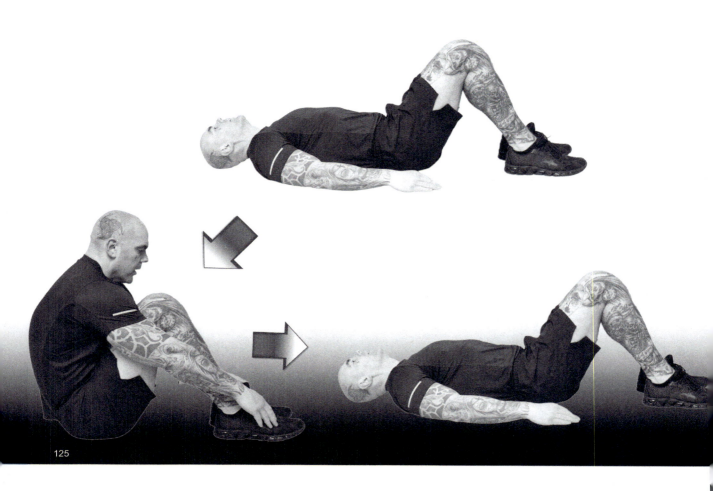

CRUNCHES

Step 1: Lie on the floor on your back.

Step 2: Lift your feet off the floor bending your knees so your shins are parallel to the floor.

Step 3: Lift your shoulders off the floor and crunch your upper body up towards your knees.

Step 4: Lower yourself back down but don't let your shoulders touch the floor keep the tension in. Then repeat.

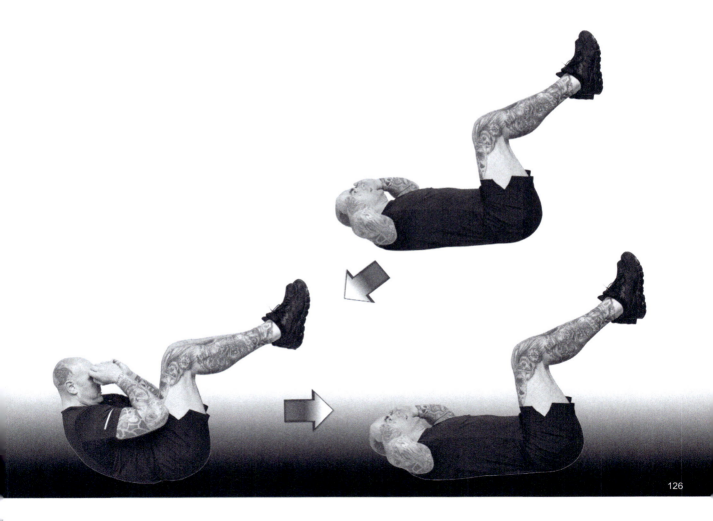

HEEL TAPS

Step 1: Lie with your back on the floor.

Step 2: Keep your knees bent and with one hand touch your heel.

Step 3: Repeat with the other hand touching the other heel. Then repeat.

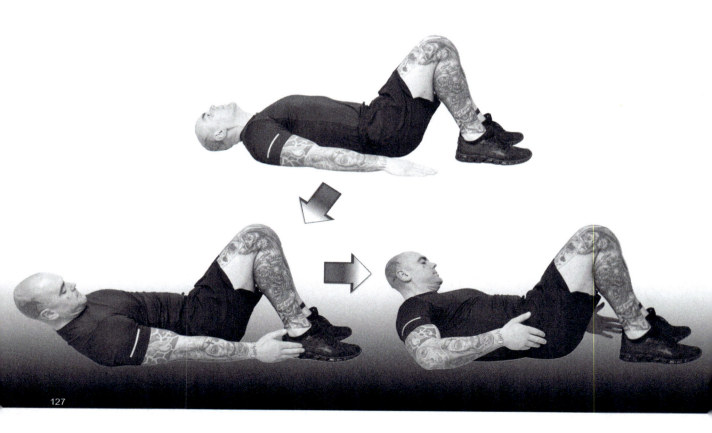

LEG RAISES

Step 1: Lie flat on your back on the floor.

Step 2: Put your hands at the bottom of your back for support and stability.

Step 3: Keep your feet together and lift them off the floor till your legs are at a 90° angle and return your legs back down but don't touch the ground, keeping the tension in. Then repeat.

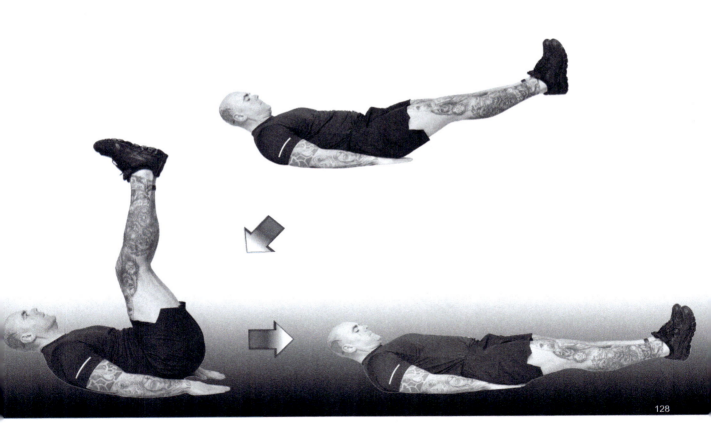

BICYCLE

Step 1: Lie on your back on the floor.

Step 2: Lift your feet off the floor so that you are in a crunch position.

Step 3: Begin pedalling as if you are riding a bike straightening your legs out as you do it. Then repeat.

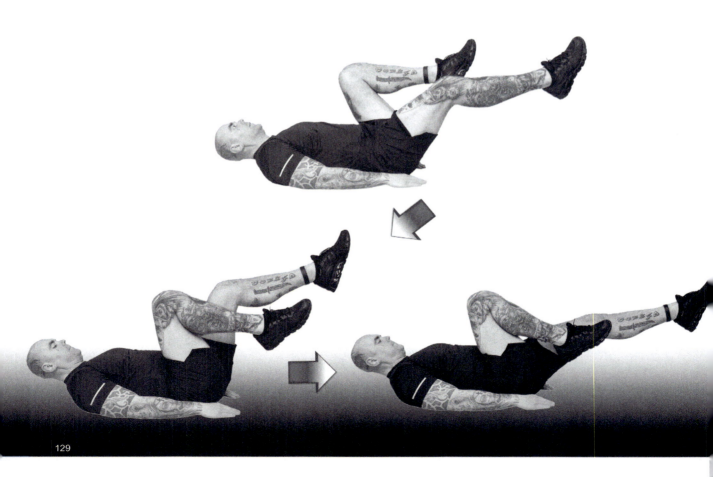

CRUNCH TWIST

Step 1: Lie on the floor with knees bent up in front of you.

Step 2: Place your hands at the side of your head with your fingertips touching your head.

Step 3: Lift your shoulders off the floor and crunch your body up touching your left knee with your right elbow then return and repeat with other side touching your right knee with your left elbow. Then repeat.

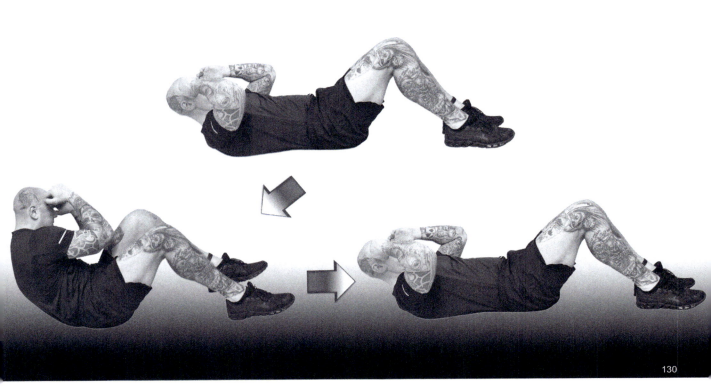

FULL PLANK

Step 1: Go down on your knees and put your hands on the floor shoulder width apart extending your arms out.

Step 2: Extend your legs out and enagage your core and keep your body stiff.

Step 3: Hold this position for as long as possible.

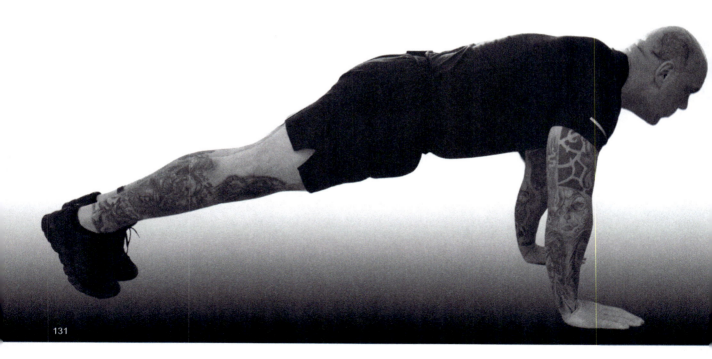

HALF PLANK

Step 1: Place your forearms on the ground and stretch your body out.

Step 2: Keep your feet together and engage your core and stay elevated of the floor.

Step 2: Hold the position keeping your head upright and core tight.

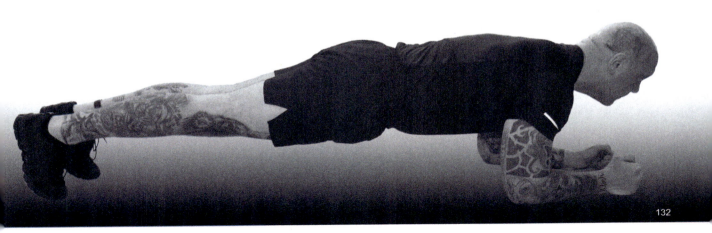

PRESS UP

Step 1: Put your hands on the ground shoulder width apart.

Step 2: Extend your legs out fully and engage your core with arms fully extended.

Step 3: Lower your chest to the floor bending your elbows and push back up to starting position. Then repeat.

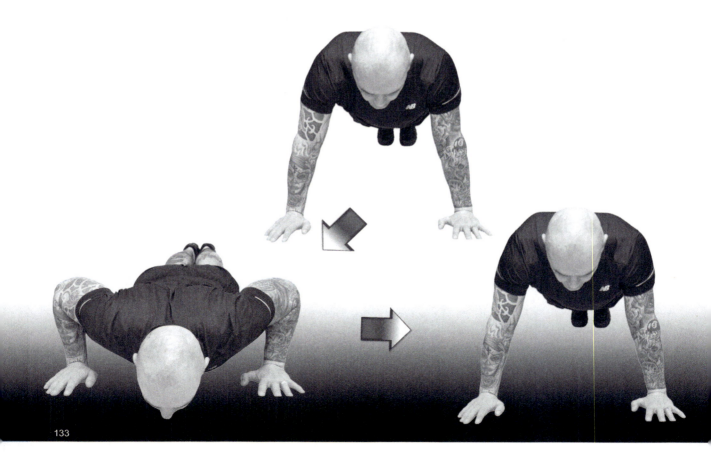

PRESS UP CLAP

Step 1: From the press up position lower your body to the floor.

Step 2: Push up explosively lift your hands off the floor and clap placing your hands back to the floor. Then repeat.

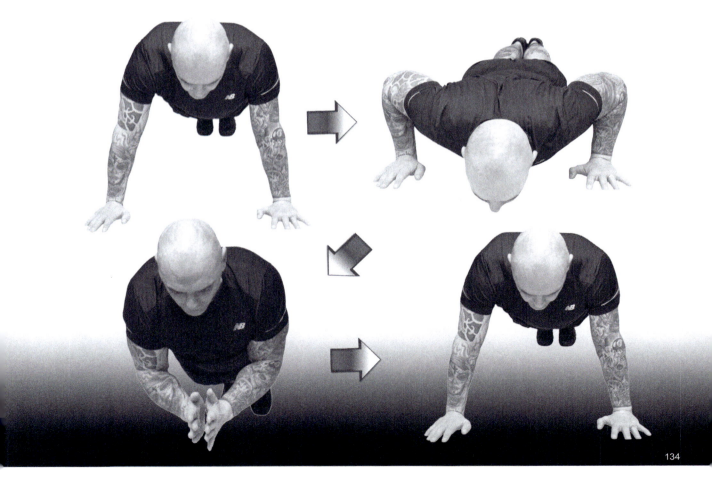

INCLINE PRESS UPS

Step 1: Place your hands on a bench or chair shoulder with a part.

Step 2: Straighten your legs out behind you lower your body down towards the bench.

Step 3: Push back up and repeat.

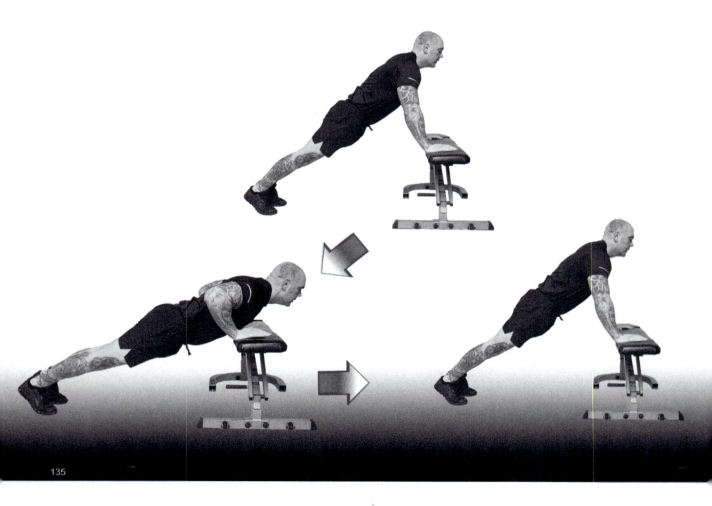

DECLINE PRESS UPS

Step 1: Place your feet together on the bench with your hands shoulder width apart.

Step 2: Lower your body towards the floor and come down till your chin is an inch of the floor.

Step 3: Push back up. Then repeat.

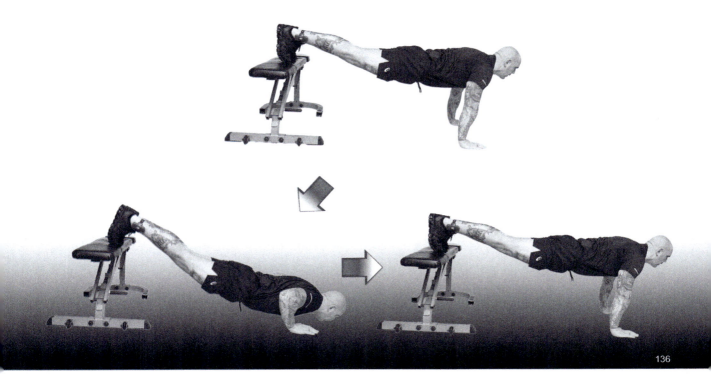

PIKE PRESS UPS

Step 1: Place your hands on the floor shoulder width apart.

Step 2: Place your feet further up with your bottom in the air.

Step 3: Keep your head down so the top of your head is facing the floor and lower your head down towards the floor, push back up. Then repeat.

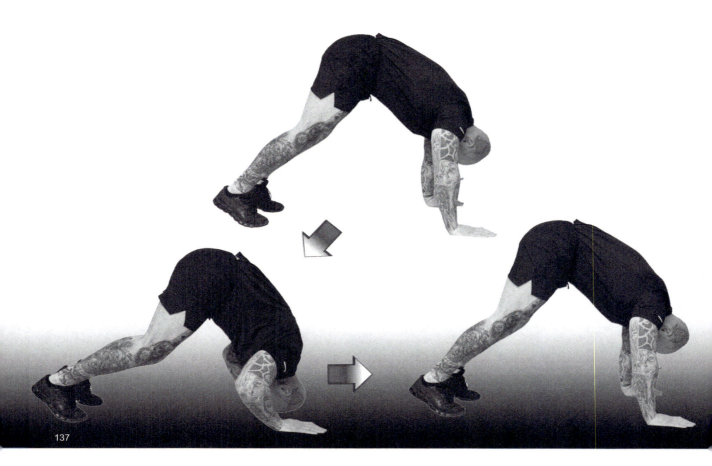

JUMPING JACKS.

Step 1: Standing upright with your feet together looking forward.

Step 2: Moving your arms and legs at the same time bring your arms out to the side and up above your head in a circular motion and slightly jump and extend your legs to shoulder width apart.

Step 3: Return your arms and legs to the starting position. Then repeat.

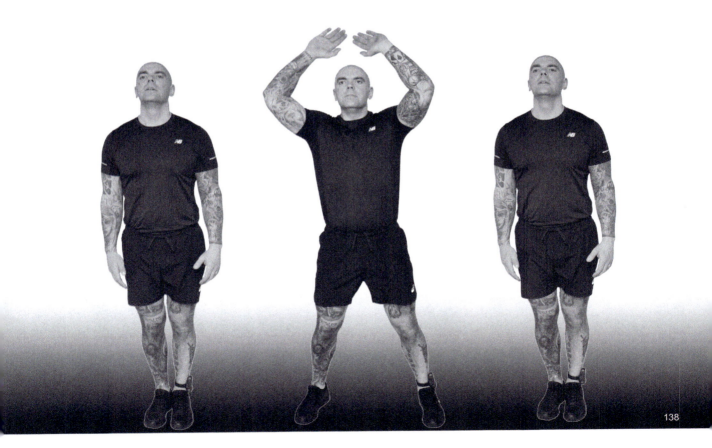

STEP UPS

Step 1: Using a chair, bench or step box, stand about a foot away from the box looking forward with your back straight step up with 1 foot and push through bringing your other leg up so you are standing on the box.

Step 2: With the first leg you used step back down and return both feet to the floor and alternate between legs every time you step up. Then repeat.

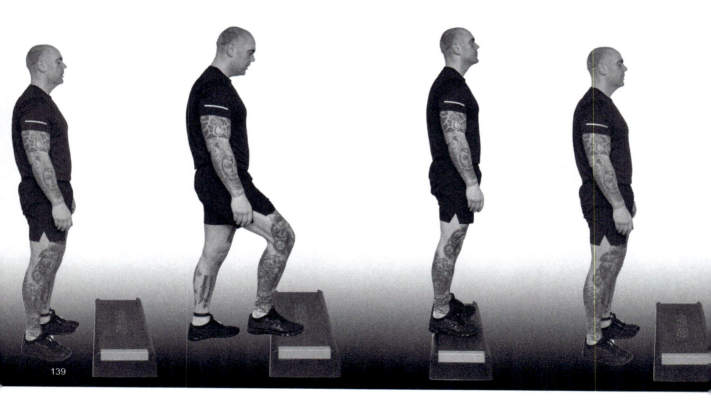

BEAR CRAWL

Step 1: Place your hands on the floor shoulder width apart and keep your body elevated.

Step 2: Move right hand forward then right leg forward placing your right knee on the outside of your elbow.

Step 3: Move your left hand forward then left leg placing your knee on the outside of your elbow.

Step 4: Repeat again keep moving forward.

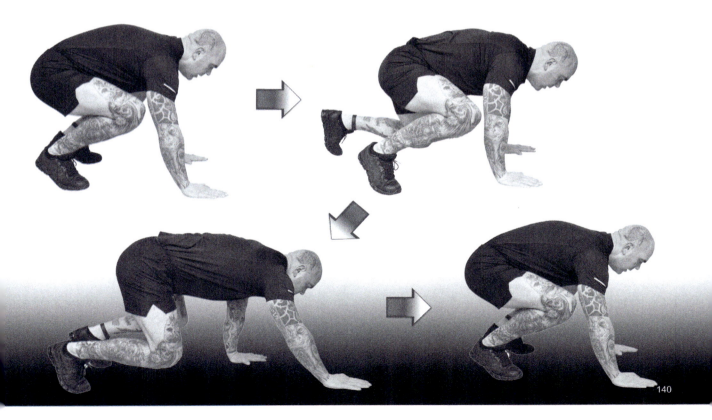

DIPS

Step 1: Holding onto a bench with your hands behind you hip width apart keep your legs straight out in front of you.

Step 2: Lower your backside down towards the floor bending your arms as you lower yourself.

Step 3: Push back up until your arms are straight. Then repeat.

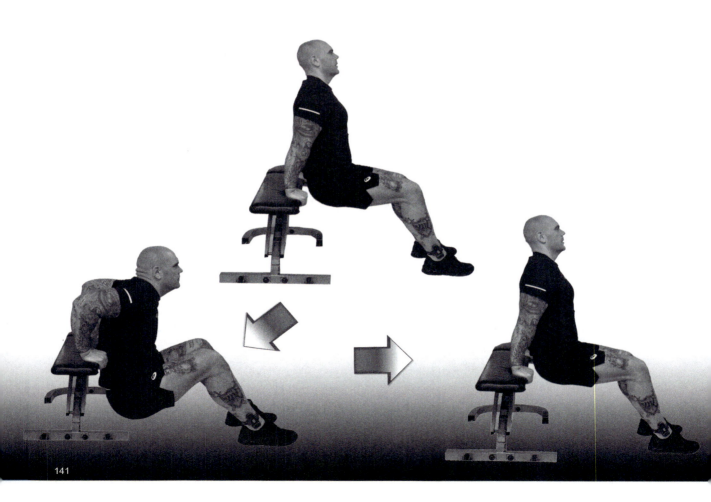

BAR DIPS

Step 1: Grip the bars parallel to your body and lift your feet of the floor and keep them elevated.

Step 2: Slowly lower your body down so that your shoulders become level with the bars.

Step 3: Push back up keeping your body stiff and extend your arms out so they are straight. Then repeat.

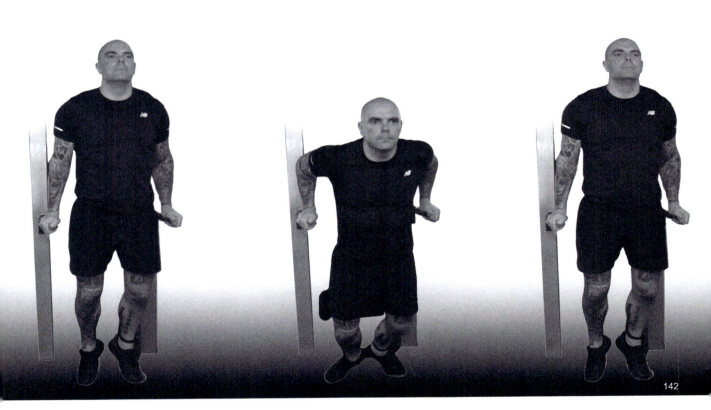

HIGH KNEES

Step 1: Stand upright facing forwards with your hands out in front of you at hip height.

Step 2: Bring your left knee up to your left hand then return to the floor landing on your tip toes.

Step 3: Do the same with your right leg bringing your knee up to your right hand before returning to the floor.

Step 4: Repeat the process landing lightly on your tip toes each time.

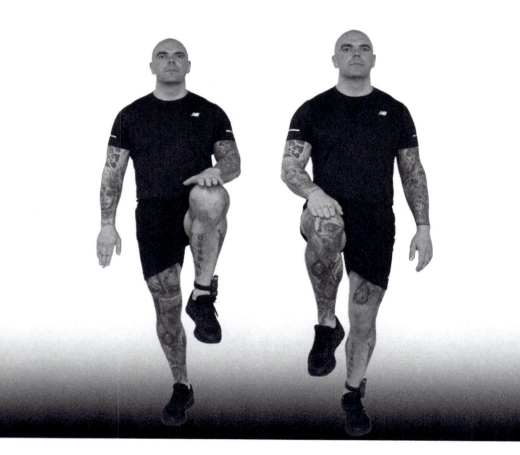

UNDER ARM PULL UPS

Step 1: Grab the bar underarm so that your hands are gripping the bar about 6 inches apart.

Step 2: Pull your body up so that your chin goes above the bar and squeeze at the top with your biceps.

Step 3: Slowly lower your body back down in a controlled manner so your arms are fully extended. Then repeat.

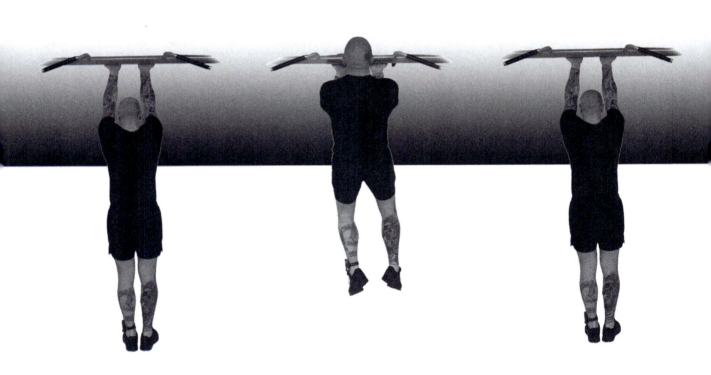

INVERTED GRIP PULL UPS

Step 1: Grab the bars on the side angle and lift your feet off the floor.

Step 2: Pull your body up lifting your chin above the bar squeezing at the top.

Step 3: Lower your body back down in a controlled manner until your arms are fully extended. Then repeat.

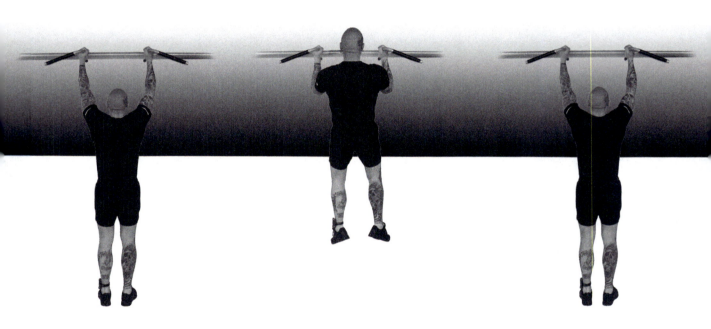

OVERARM PULL UPS

Step 1: Grab the bar overarm just wider than shoulder width apart and lift your feet off the floor.

Step 2: Pull your body up lifting your chin above the bar and squeezing at the top.

Step 3: Lower your body back down in a controlled manner until your arms are fully extended. Then repeat.

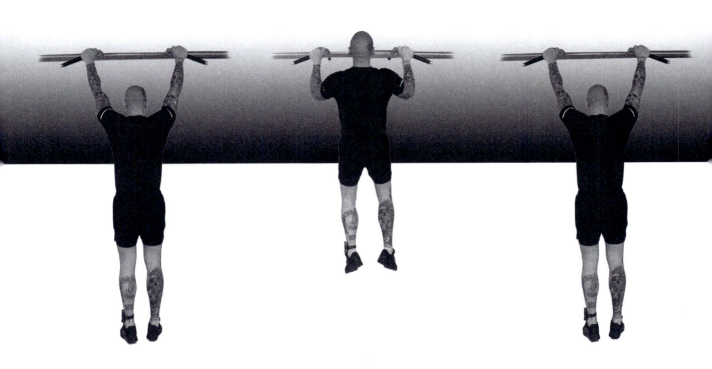

UNDER ARM ROWS

Step 1: Holding onto a bar or whatever is available lean back until your arms are fully extended.

Step 2: Pull your body up towards the bar squeezing your back as you reach the top.

Step 3: Lower yourself back down keeping a hold of the bar. Then repeat.

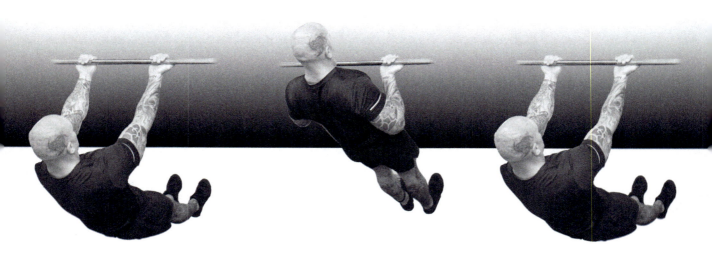

DORSAL RAISE

Step 1: Lie on the floor face down with your arms relaxed at your sides.

Step 2: Raise your upper body of the floor lifting your shoulders off the floor feeling the squeeze in your lower back.

Step 3: Lower yourself back down then repeat.

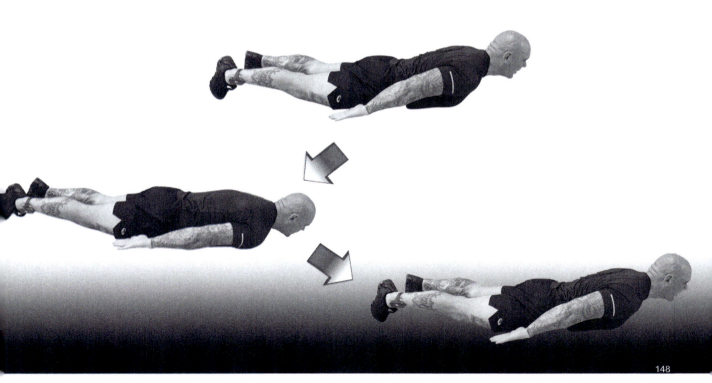

WEIGHTLIFTING EXERCISES

These exercises are to be performed with weights ideally in a gym. The reason we do weightlifting exercises is to enhance our muscles and ultimately get bigger and stronger. Depending on how much you lift and how many times you lift the weights will give you different results.

I will now explain all the weightlifting exercises that I have done and will explain step by step for each of the exercises.

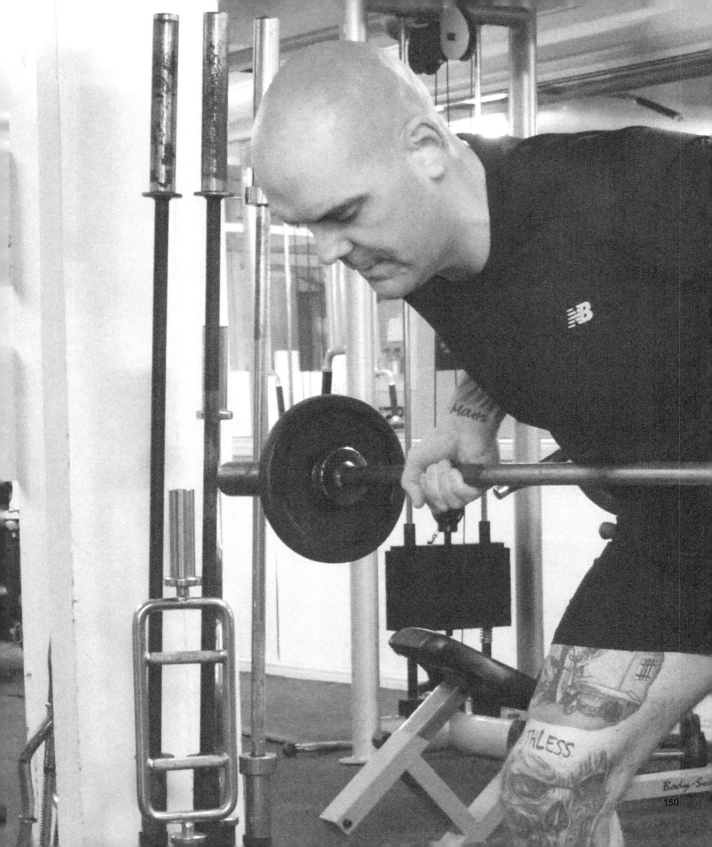

SECTION ONE: CHEST EXERCISES

The following exercises target the pectoral muscles also known as your pecs and chest muscles. The pectoral muscle has three different areas you need to exercise, even though this is one muscle we need to target all three different areas to get the full effect.

The three areas are upper, middle and lower. Upper is incline bench exercises, middle is on flat bench exercises and lower is decline bench exercises.

BENCH PRESS

Step 1: Lie on a bench and place your feet firmly on the floor.

Step 2: Grab the bar just slightly wider than shoulder width apart and lift the bar and hold it with your arms fully extended.

Step 3: Lower the bar down to your chest hold it for a second then push it back through until your arms are fully extended again keeping your feet firmly on the floor and your back on the bench. Then repeat.

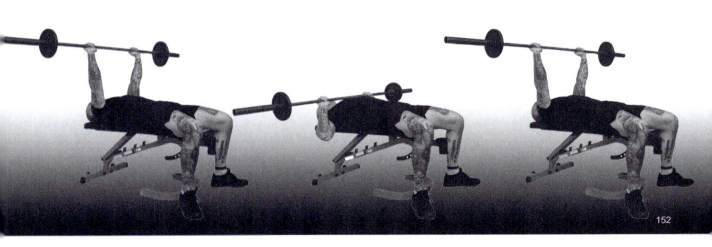

INCLINE BENCH PRESS

Step 1: Lie on a bench that is set at an inclined angle.

Step 2: Grab the bar just slightly wider than shoulder width apart.

Step 3: Lift the bar and hold it with your arms fully extended.

Step 4: Come just below your chin and hold for a second before pushing back up using your legs to keep your feet firm on the floor and your back to push through up into your arms and chest and fully extend your arms. Then repeat.

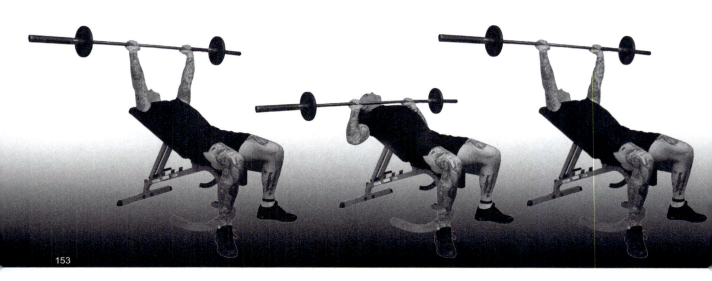

DECLINE BENCH PRESS

Step 1: Lie back on a decline bench and hook your feet under the support bars.

Step 2: Grab the bar just slightly wider than shoulder width apart.

Step 3: Lift the bar hold it out with your arms fully extended.

Step 4: Lower the bar down to your chest, hold it for a second then push back through using your triceps and squeezing your chest as you fully extend your arms. Then repeat.

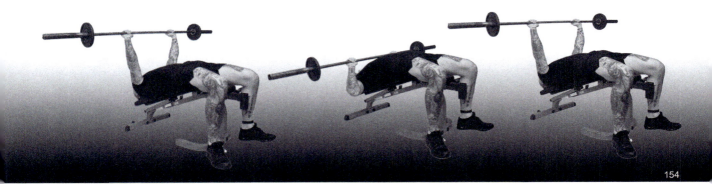

DUMBBELL BENCH PRESS

Step 1: Holding the dumbbells lie back on the bench and hold the dumbbells with your arms fully extended.

Step 2: Lower the dumbbells to your chest shoulder width apart and push back up until your arms are fully extended. Then repeat.

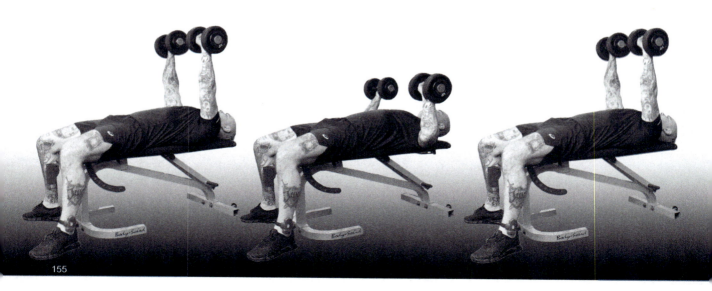

DUMBBELL FLYES

Step 1: Holding the dumbbells lie back on the bench and hold the dumbbells with your arms fully extended.

Step 2: At the same time lower the dumbbells outwards keeping your elbows slightly bent and lower until your arms are in line with your chest then lift the dumbbells back up and squeeze at the top. Then repeat.

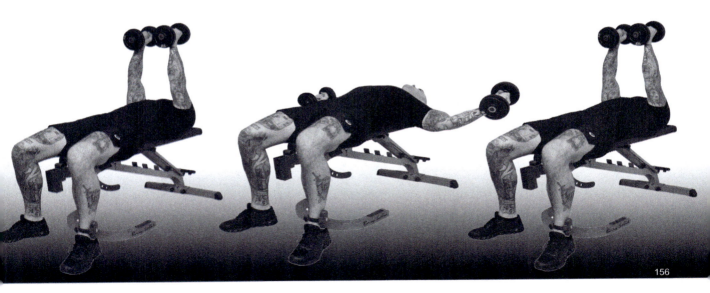

CABLE FLYES

Step 1: Grab the handles and stand with your back straight and push your chest out with one foot in front of the other for balance, lean forward and hold the cables at chest height.

Step 2: Keep your elbows slightly bent and pull the cables out so your hands come together and squeeze.

Step 3: In a controlled manner let your arms lower the weights so your arms return back to the starting position. Then repeat.

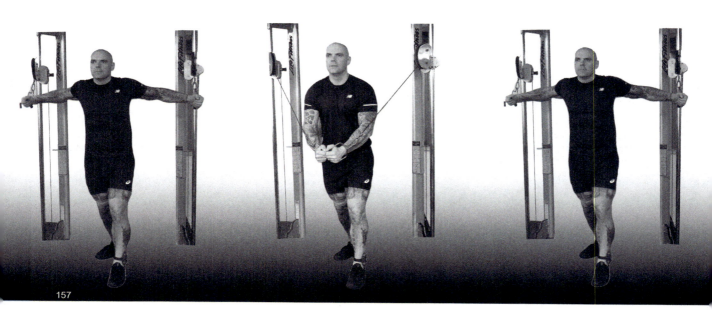

PECK DECK MACHINE

Step 1: Sit on the seat and grab the handles.

Step 2: Push the handles and feel your chest squeeze as you push them together until the bars touch then return to start position and repeat.

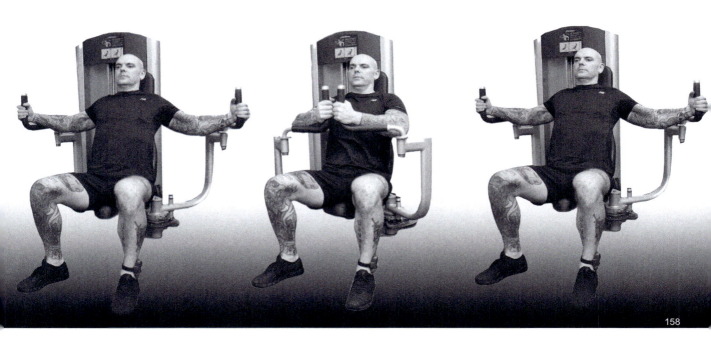

SECTION TWO: BICEPS EXERCISES

The following exercises target your bicep muscles also known as your Bi's. All bicep exercises are performed by doing a curling movement. The bicep is a muscle on the front part of the upper arm. The bicep is made up of a long head and a short head. The long head runs along the outside of the upper arm and gives the appearance of length and the short head is closest to the body on the inner arm and gives the appearance of fullness and roundness. All the exercises target both areas of the biceps.

BARBELL CURLS

Step 1: Grab the bar hip width apart underarm and hold it in front of you keeping your back straight and knees slightly bent so they are loose, keep your elbows tucked in.

Step 2: Lift the bar up towards your chin keeping your elbows tucked in so you are only moving your forearms and squeeze at the top.

Step 3: Slowly lower the bar back down so that your arms are extended but slightly bent then repeat.

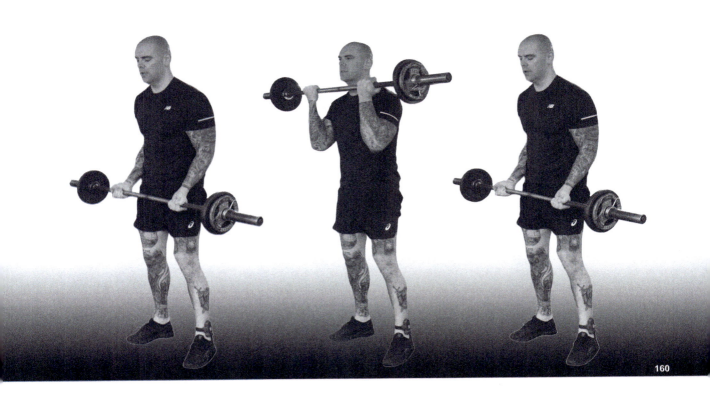

EZ BAR CURLS

Step 1: Grab the bar hip width apart underarm and hold it in front of you keeping your back straight and knees slightly bent so they are loose, keep your elbows tucked in.

Step 2: Lift the bar up towards your chin keeping your elbows tucked in so you are only moving your forearms and squeeze at the top.

Step 3: Slowly lower the bar back down so that your arms are extended but slightly bent then repeat.

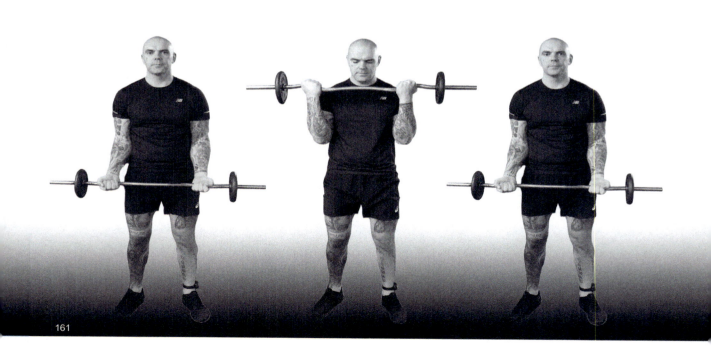

CLOSE GRIP EZ BAR CURLS

Step 1: Grab the bar closegrip so your hands are nearly touching side by side.

Step 2: Lift the bar up towards your chin keeping your elbows tucked in so you are only moving your forearms and squeeze at the top.

Step 3: Slowly lower the bar back down so that your arms are extended but slightly bent then repeat.

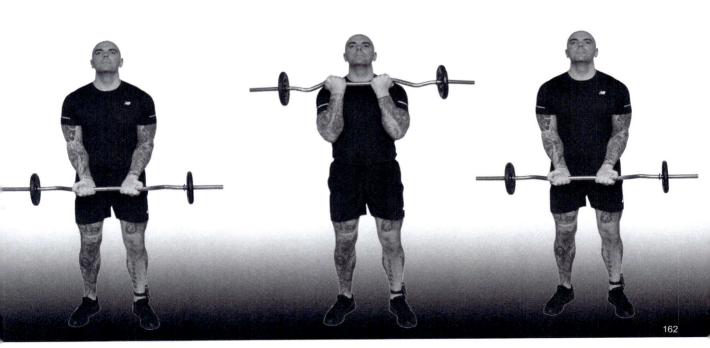

DUMBBELL CURL

Step 1: Hold the dumbbells at the side of your legs with your knuckles facing outwards, keep your back straight and knees slightly bent so they are loose and keep your elbows tucked in.

Step 2: Lift the dumbbells up towards your shoulders then turn them so your knuckles are now facing down instead of out and squeeze at the top.

Step 3: Lower the dumbbells back down turning your wrist so your knuckles are facing outwards then repeat.

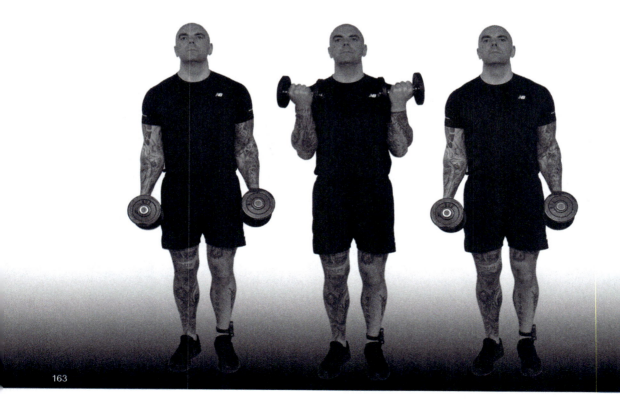

HAMMER CURL

Step 1: Hold the dumbbells at the side of your legs with your knuckles facing outwards, keep your back straight and knees slightly bent so they are loose and keep your elbows tucked in.

Step 2: Lift the dumbbells up towards your shoulders and keep your knuckles facing outwards as you squeeze at the top keeping your elbows tucked in.

Step 3: Slowly lower the dumbbells back down till your arms are extended, hold then repeat.

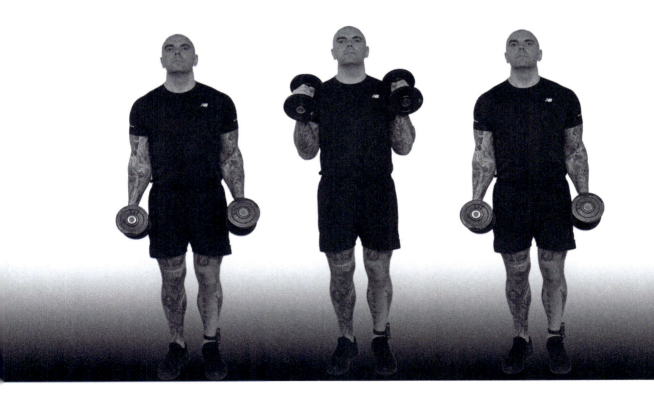

SECTION THREE:

TRICEP EXERCISES

The following exercises target your triceps muscles also known as tri's. The triceps is a muscle on the back of the upper arm and consists of 3 heads. These are the medial, lateral and long head. All of the following exercise target these areas.

The medial head is on the middle of the back portion of the upper arm, the lateral head is the outer part of your triceps and the long head is the largest part of your triceps running down the back of your arm. All of these exercise will target all 3 heads.

CLOSE GRIP BENCH PRESS

Step 1: Lie back on a bench and grab the bar slightly closer than shoulder width apart (or a 6 inch gap in between hands) and hold the bar out with your arms fully extended.

Step 2: Lower the bar to your chest then push back through with your triceps keeping your feet firmly on the floor and your back on the bench until your arms are fully extended. Then repeat.

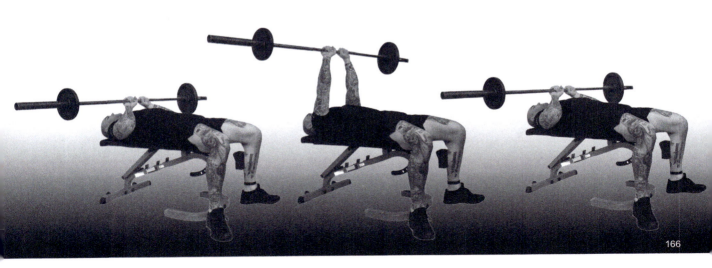

T BAR CABLE PUSH DOWN

Step 1: Grab the bar firmly with your elbows bent and slightly bend your knees and keep your back straight.

Step 2: Push the bar down so that your arms are fully extended out then slowly bring the bar back up bending your elbows as you do. Then repeat.

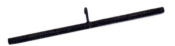

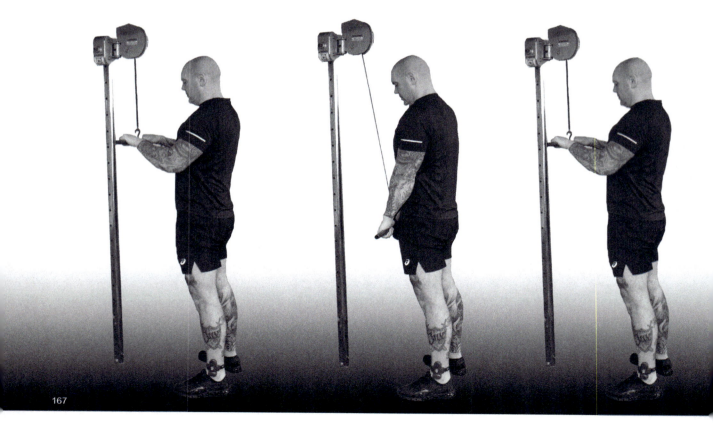

ROPE PUSH DOWN

Step 1: Grab the rope at chest height and hold it so your hands are nearly touching.

Step 2: Pull the rope down towards your hips and at the same time pushing the rope pull it outwards until your arms are fully extended and squeeze before returning to the start position. Then repeat.

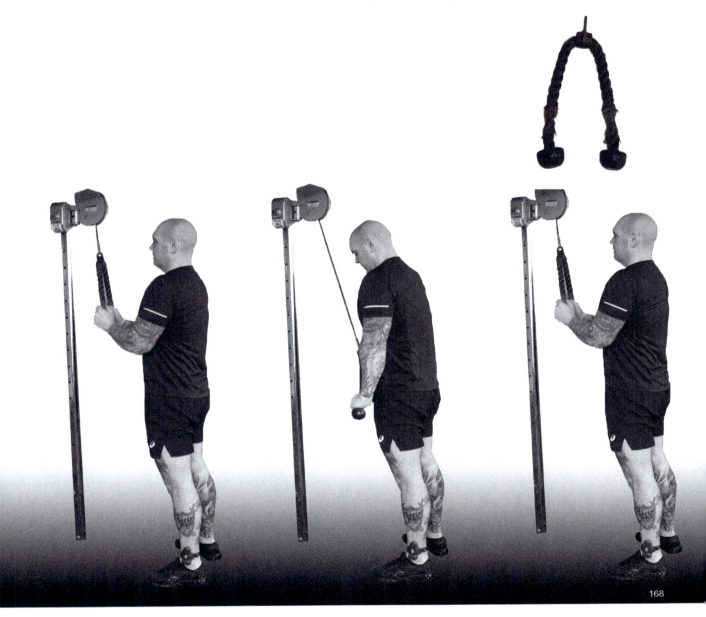

V-BAR PUSH DOWN

Step 1: Grab the bar firmly with your arms bent and slightly bend your knees and keep your back straight.

Step 2: Push the bar down so that your arms are fully extended out then slowly bring the bar back up bending your arms and

elbows as you do. Then repeat.

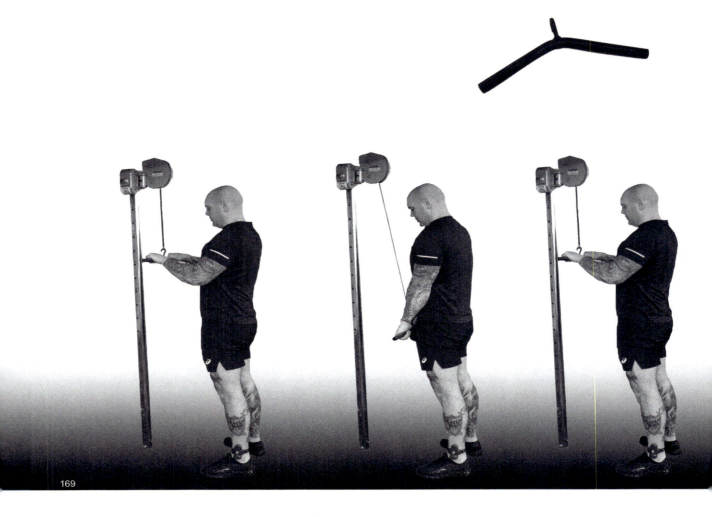

SKULL CRUSHES

Step 1: Lying on a flat bench hold the bar with your hands next to each other, hold the bar out with your arms fully extended.

Step 2: Slowly lower the bar bending your elbows, lower the bar towards your head coming a few inches from the top of your head.

Step 3: Hold then push back through until your arms are fully extended. Then repeat.

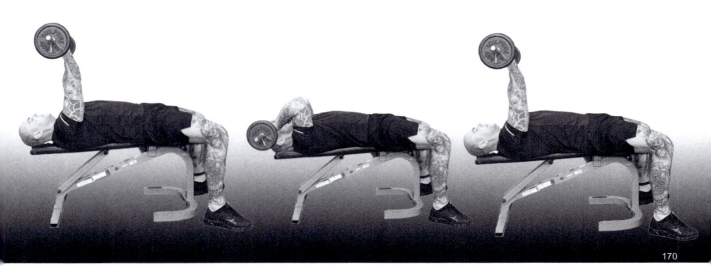

DUMBBELL TRICEP EXTENSION

Step 1: Lean on a bench placing your hand on the bench.

Step 2: With your other arm extend the dumbbell out behind you until your arm is fully extended.

Step 3: Lower the dumbbell back to starting position. Then repeat.

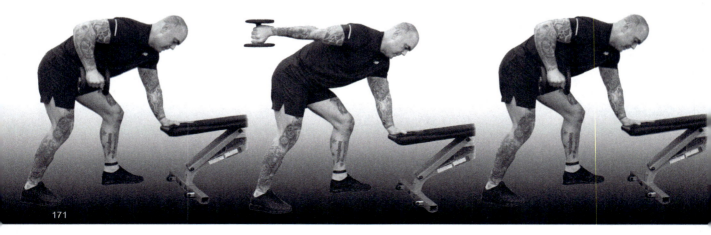

TRICEP SKI

Step 1: Stand with a dumbbell in each hand.

Step 2: Lean forward keeping your back flat and bending your knees. Lift your elbows up so they are at your sides.

Step 3: At the same time push the dumbbells out behind you straightening your arms out feeling the squeeze in your triceps.

Step 4: Slowly lower the dumbbells back to starting position then repeat.

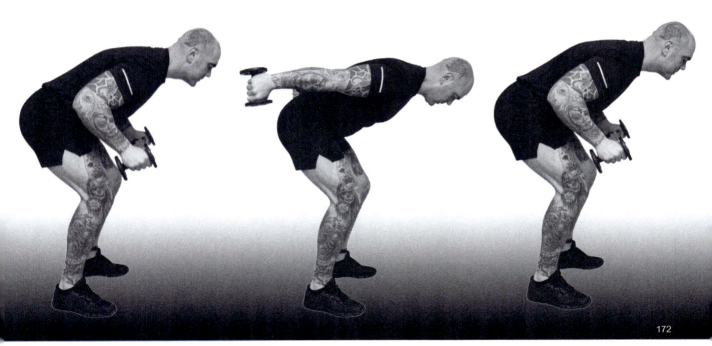

BEHIND NECK DUMBBELL EXTENSION

Step 1: Standing upright with a dumbbell in one hand hold the dumbbell behind your head with your elbow pointing upwards.

Step 2: Keep your arm and elbow straight push up and extend your arm out fully.

Step 3: Lower the dumbbell back to start position. Then repeat.

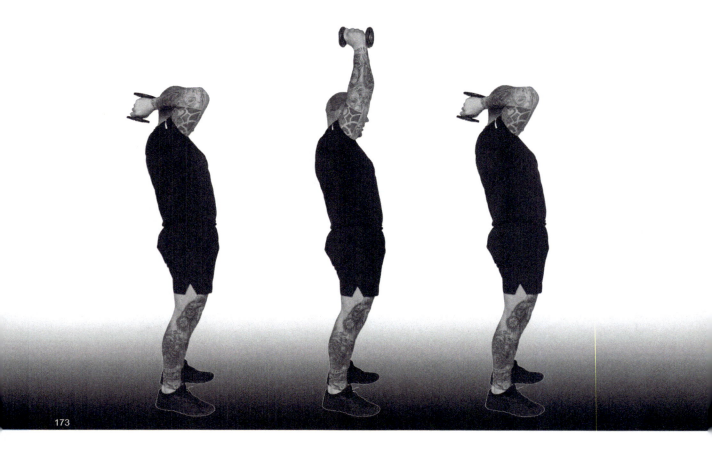

SECTION FOUR: BACK EXERCISES

The following exercises target the back muscles. The back muscles consist of lower back and upper back. The lower back muscles are the erector spinae that run from the bottom of your back to the top either side of your spine. The upper back muscles are your lattissimus dorsi also known as your lats, this is the largest muscle in your back which runs from just beneath your armpit to the centre of your back.

Then you have the rhomboids that cover the area between your shoulder blades. There is also your trapezius also known as your traps which runs from the top of your neck to the edge of your shoulders and goes down the top of your back and narrows down the centre. The deadlift is the best exercise for lower back and all the other exercises target your upper back muscles. The shrugs target your trap muscles.

DEADLIFT

Step 1: Stand over the bar with your shins nearly touching the bar, with your feet hip width apart.

Step 2: Bend down with your knees bent keeping your back flat grab the bar shoulder width apart.

Step 3: Lower your buttocks down so your thighs are parallel with the floor and pull up with your back so your arms are fully extended and at the same time pushing through with your legs lift the bar off the floor until you are standing upright keeping your back flat.

Step 4: Slowly lower the bar back down to the floor bending your knees as you lower. Then repeat.

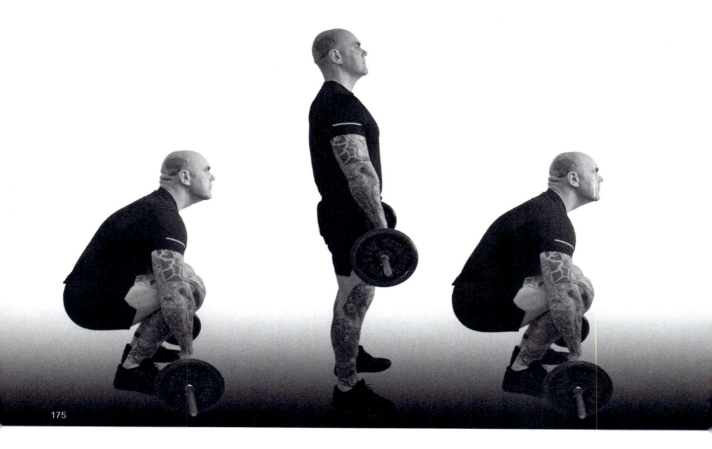

WIDE GRIP LAT PULLDOWN

Step 1: Sitting down with your legs tucked under the pads grip the bar near the end so you have a wide grip.

Step 2: Keep your feet firmly on the floor as you lean back slightly and pull the bar down to your chest squeezing your back muscles as you do this.

Step 3: Slowly let the bar go back up. Then repeat.

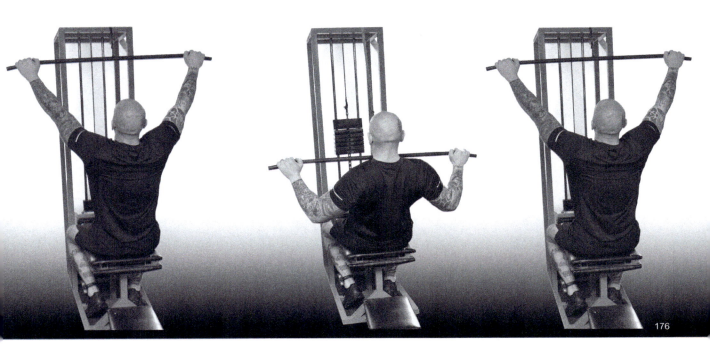

CLOSE GRIP LAT PULLDOWN

Step 1: Grab the close grip bar and sit down tucking your legs under the support pads.

Step 2: Keep your feet firmly on the floor as you lean back slightly and pull the bar down to your chest squeezing your back muscles as you do this.

Step 3: Slowly let the bar go back up. Then repeat.

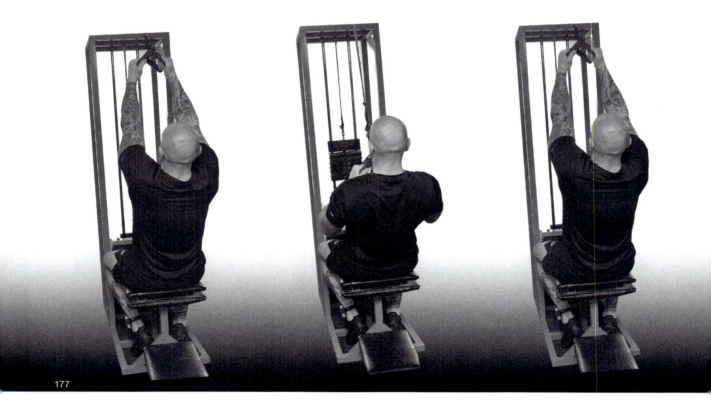

UNDER ARM LAT PULLDOWN

Step 1: Grip the bar underarm about 6 inches apart and sit down tucking your legs under the support bar.

Step 2: Keep your feet firmly on the floor as you lean back slightly with your arms fully extended out and pull the bar down to your chest squeezing your back muscles as you do this.

Step 3: Slowly let the bar go back up. Then repeat.

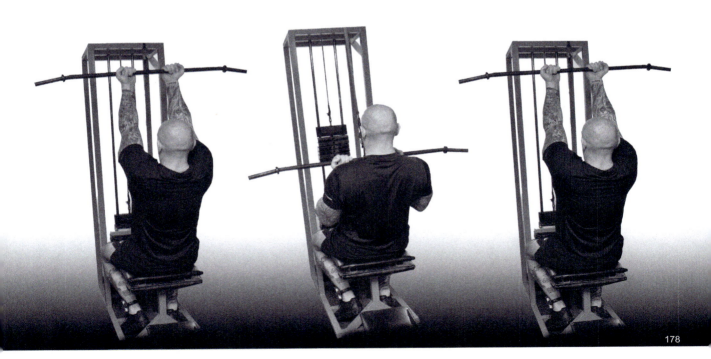

BARBELL BENT-OVER ROWS

Step 1: Standing above the bar grip the bar underarm shoulder width apart, bending your knees and keeping your back flat.

Step 2: Lift the bar of the floor with your arms extended out in front of you.

Step 3: Pull the bar up towards the bottom of your chest feeling the squeeze as you pull it up.

Step 4: Slowly lower the bar down to the floor keeping your back flat as you do this. Then repeat.

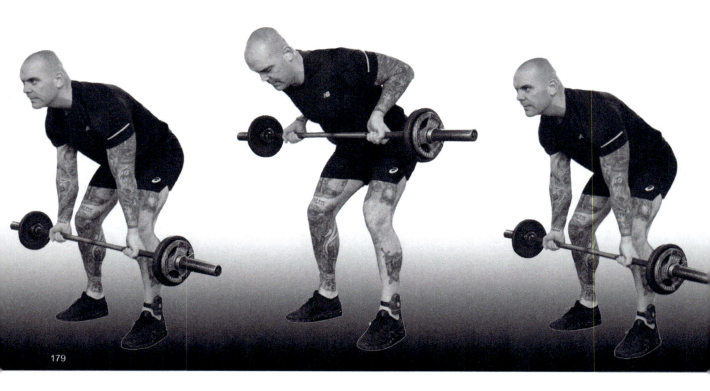

ONE ARM DUMBBELL ROWS

Step 1: Place your left knee on the bench and lean forward on the bench keeping your opposite foot firmly on the floor and keep your back flat.

Step 2: Lift the dumbbell of the floor and keep your arm fully extended.

Step 3: Pull the dumbbell up to your chest feeling your side lats squeeze at the top.

Step 4: Slowly lower the dumbbell back down. Then repeat.

Step 5: Repeat with your opposite side after you have finished your reps.

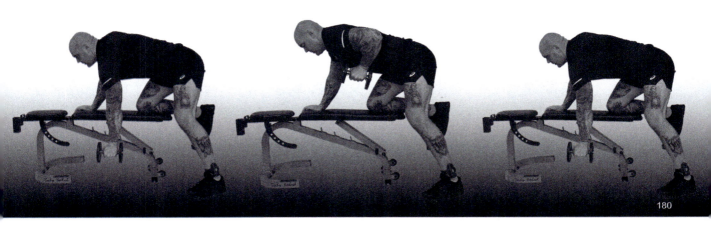

SEATED ROWS

Step 1: Sitting on the machine grip the handles and engage your back keeping it straight.

Step 2: Pull the handles and feel the squeeze in your side lats and back then slowly lower back to start position. Then repeat.

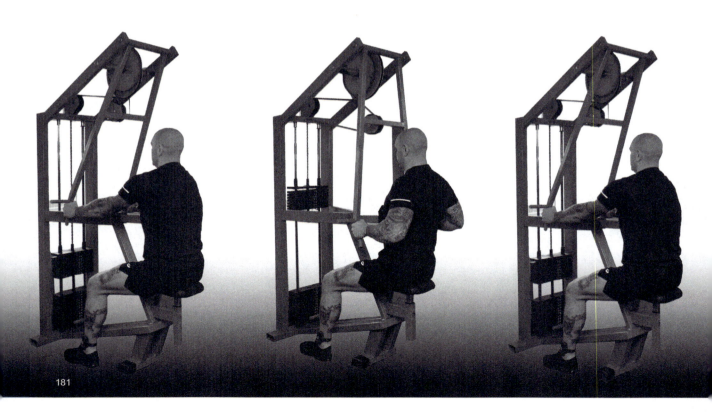

SECTION FIVE: SHOULDER EXERCISES

The following exercises target your deltoid muscles also known as your shoulders. Your shoulders are made up of 3 heads.

The anterior which is the front delt, the medial which is the side delt and posterior which is the rear delt. The pressing exercises target all your deltoids. The side exercises target your side delts and the bent over exercises target your rear delts.

KETTLE BELL SWING

Step 1: Bend down keeping your knees bent and back flat and grab the kettlebell with both hands.

Step 2: Stand upright then let the kettlebell swing in-between your legs as you squat down slightly and bend forwards keeping your back flat at all times.

Step 3: Swing the kettlebell up in front of you to shoulder height then lower back down and repeat.

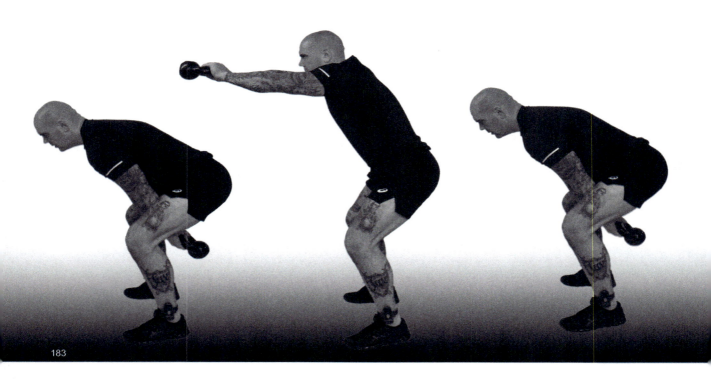

STANDING BARBELL PRESS

Step 1: Lift the bar off the floor and hold the weight in front of your shoulders, keep your knees loose and your back straight, stand with feet hip width apart for balance and support.

Step 2: Push the weight up above your head until your arms are fully extended.

Step 3: Lower the weight back down to your shoulders in a controlled manner. Then repeat.

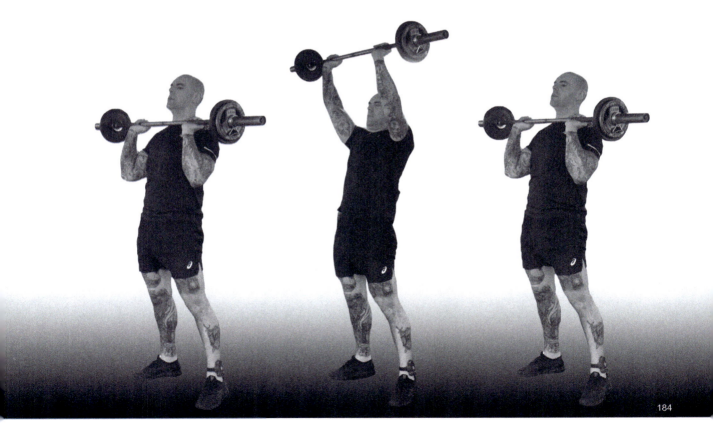

SEATED DUMBBELL PRESS

Step 1: Sit on an upright bench and pick the dumbbells off the floor and sit back and lift the dumbbells up to your shoulders.

Step 2: Push the dumbbells up until your arms are fully extended and this is the starting point.

Step 3: Keeping your feet firmly on the floor and your back pressed against the bench, lower the weight to your shoulders.

Step 4: Push back through using your legs, back and arms to drive the weight back up to the starting point. Then repeat.

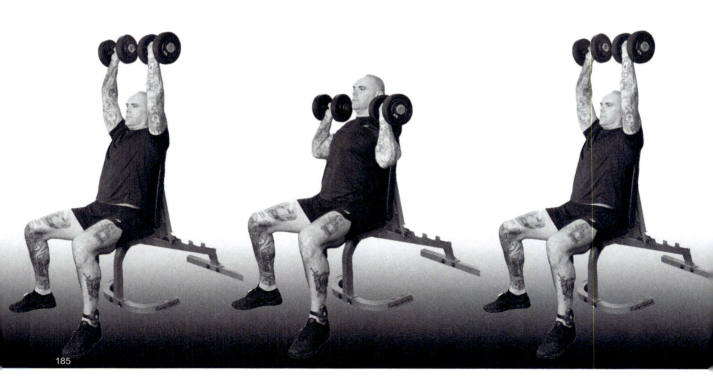

SMITH MACHINE PRESS

Step 1: Sitting on an upright angle make sure the bar is in line with the top of your chest just in front of your chin, grab the bar shoulder width apart and keep your feet firmly planted on the floor.

Step 2: Lift the bar and hold for a second.

Step 3: Lower the weight down to the top of your chest.

Step 4: Push through using your legs, engage your back and using your arms as you push up, push the bar back up to the starting position. Then repeat.

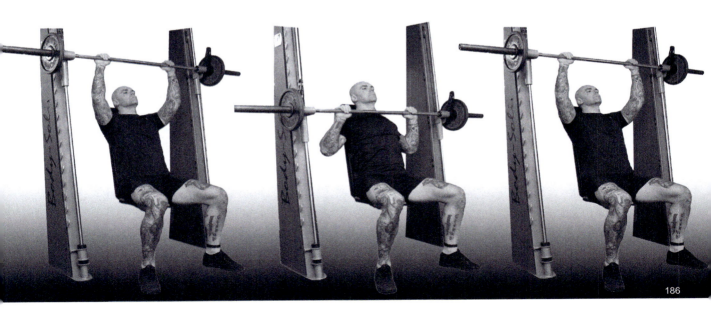

UPRIGHT ROWS (close grip)

Step 1: Lift the bar off the floor with your hands nearly touching and stand upright with your feet hip width apart.

Step 2: Hold the bar in front of you with your arms fully extended.

Step 3: Slightly bend your knees as you pull the bar up toward your chin, feeling your traps squeeze as you get to the top.

Step 4: Slowly lower the bar back down till your arms are fully extended and the bar is resting at your thighs. Then repeat.

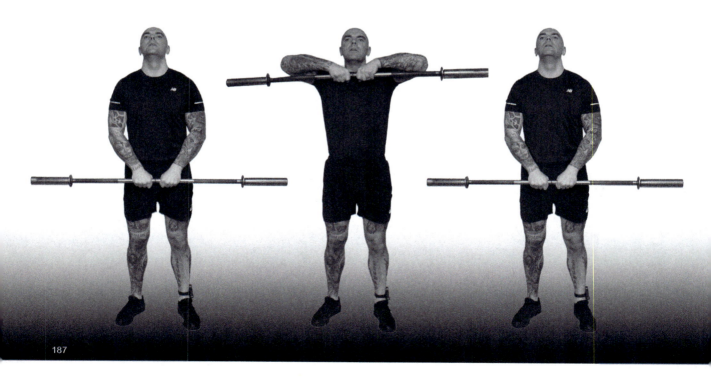

UPRIGHT ROWS (wide grip)

Step 1: Lift the bar off the floor with your hands shoulder width apart and stand upright with your feet hip width apart.

Step 2: Hold the bar in front of you with your arms fully extended.

Step 3: Slightly bend your knees as you pull the bar up toward your chin stopping as you get just below your chin feeling your traps squeeze as you get to the top.

Step 4: Slowly lower the bar back down until your arms are fully extended and the bar is resting at your thighs. Then repeat.

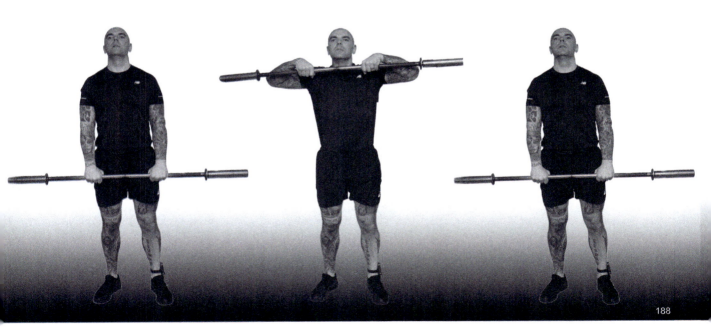

SHRUGS WITH BARBELL

Step 1: Hold the bar in front of you with the bar resting at your thighs.

Step 2: With your arms fully extended in front of you shrug your shoulders up towards your ears and squeeze at the top.

Step 3: Lower the bar back down. Then repeat.

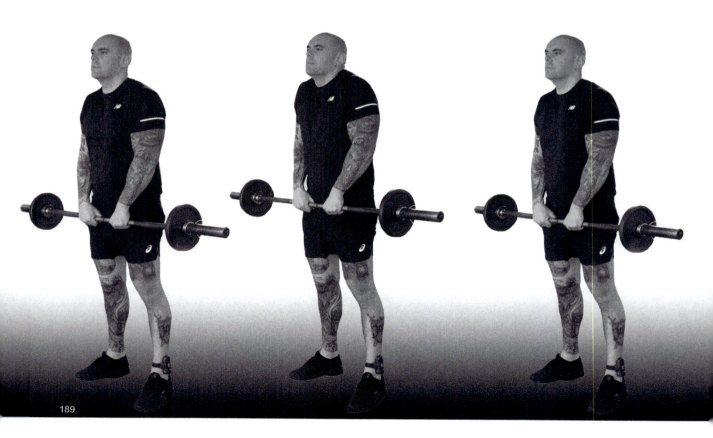

SHRUGS WITH DUMBBELLS

Step 1: Hold the dumbbells at the side of your thighs and keep your back straight and knees loose.

Step 2: With your arms fully extended shrug your shoulders up towards your ears and squeeze at the top.

Step 3: Lower your shoulders back down. Then repeat.

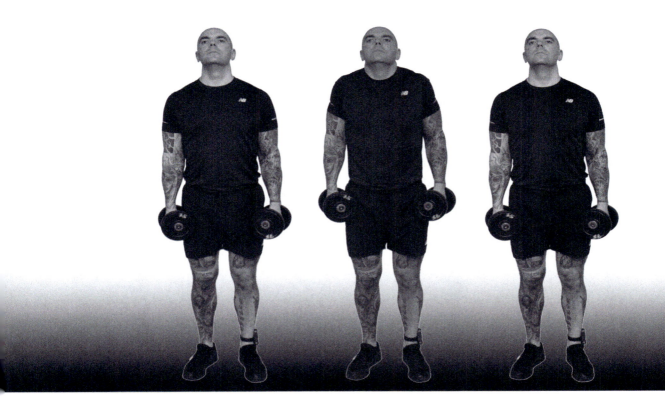

FRONT RAISES

Step 1: Hold the dumbbells with your arms fully extended in front of you resting the dumbbells on your thighs with your feet hip width apart.

Step 2: With your knees slightly bent lift one of the dumbbells upwards and outwards up to shoulder height then slowly lower it back down.

Step 3: Repeat on the other side then keep alternating. Then repeat.

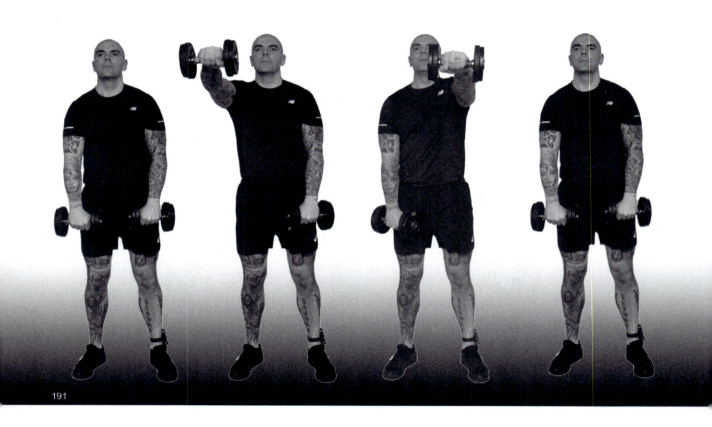

SIDE RAISES

Step 1: Hold the dumbbells at the side of your legs with your arms fully extended and your feet hip width apart.

Step 2: Keeping your back straight and knees loose lift the dumbbells at the same time outwards from the side, keeping your arms locked out up to shoulder height. Lower the dumbbells back down. Then repeat.

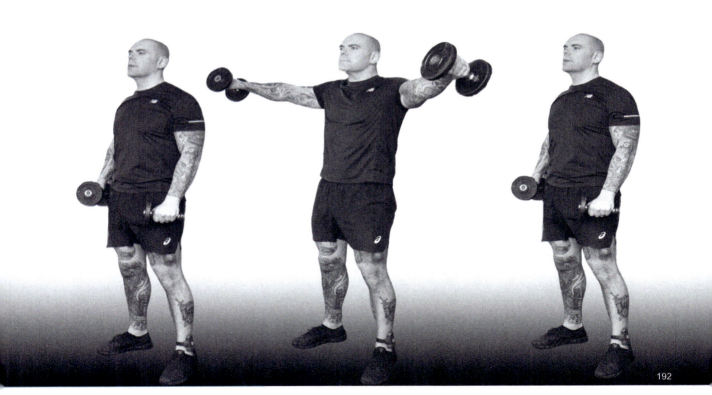

HIGH PULLS

Step 1: Standing over the bar bend down and grip the bar shoulder width apart, keeping your back flat and knees bent.

Step 2: Using your legs, back, arms and shoulders explosively pull the bar up in front of you up to your head height.

Step 3: Lower the bar back to the ground. Then repeat.

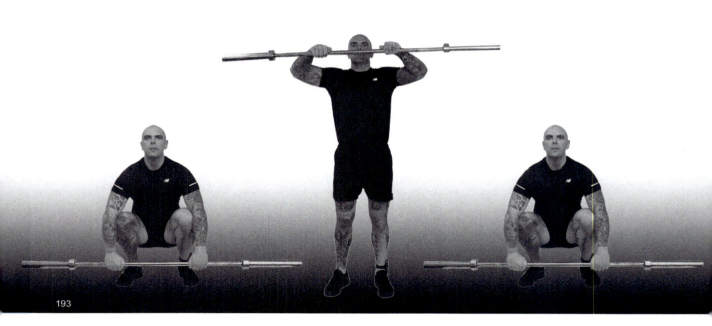

CABLE SIDE RAISES

Step 1: Using one hand grip the handle and pull the cable up from the side of your leg, standing with feet hip width apart.

Step 2: Keeping your arm locked out lift the weight outwards up to shoulder height.

Step 3: Lower the weight back down to the side of your leg. Then repeat.

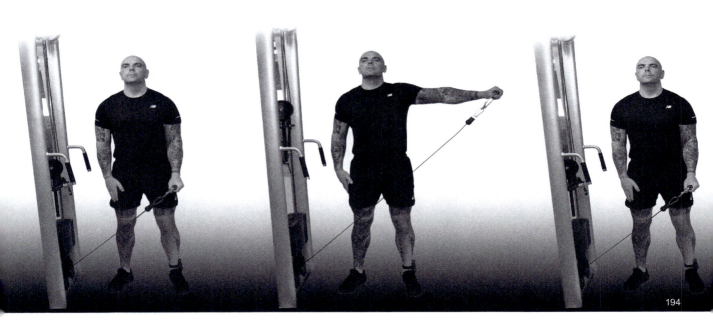

BENT OVER CABLE SIDE RAISES

Step 1: Grab the handle and bend forward placing your other hand on your knee for support.

Step 2: Pull the cable out to the side to about shoulder height.

Step 3: Lower the cable back down so your arm is vertical keeping the tension in. Then repeat.

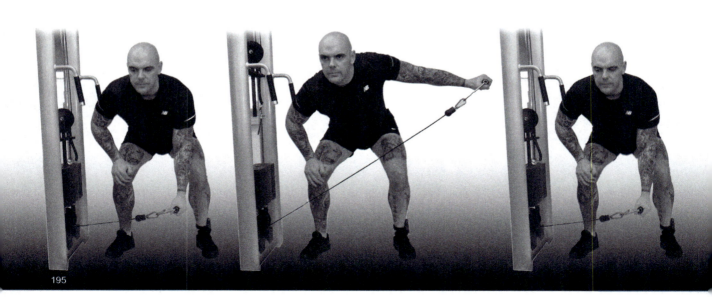

BENT OVER SIDE RAISES

Step 1: Sitting on the edge of a bench hold the dumbbells and lean forward so your chest is touching your legs and the dumbbells are under your legs.

Step 2: Bend your elbows and at the same time lift the dumbbells up and out to your sides feeling the squeeze at the top.

Step 3: Slowly lower the dumbbells back down. Then repeat.

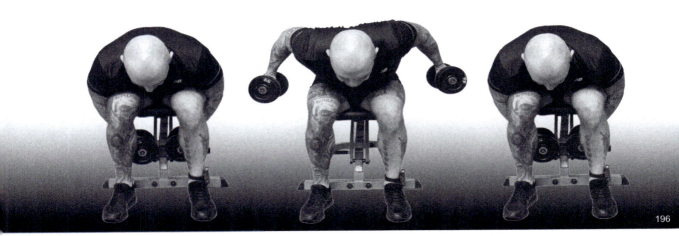

POWER CLEAN AND PRESS

Step 1: Standing over the bar bend down and grip the bar shoulder width apart keeping your back flat.

Step 2: In one motion pull the bar off the floor using your legs, back, arms and shoulders up towards your chin bending your elbows and bringing your forearms in holding the bar at shoulder height.

Step 3: Keep your knees loose and back straight, push the bar up and lock your arms out.

Step 4: Lower the bar back down to your shoulders.

Step 5: Flip the bar back over and lower it down to your waist.

Step 6: Bend your knees as you lower the bar back down to the floor keeping your back flat as you do this.

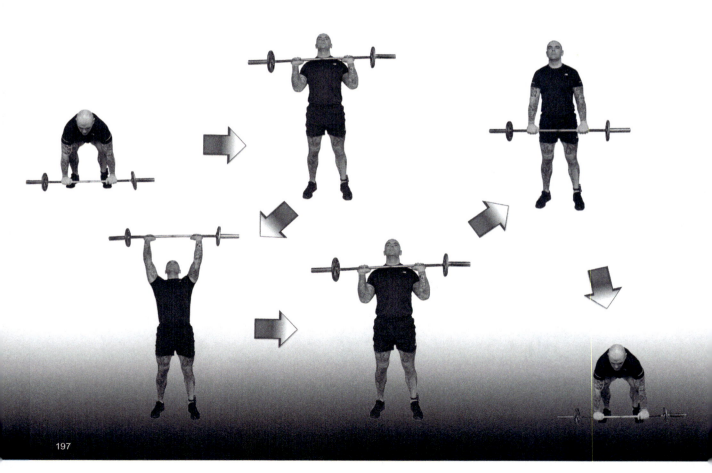

SECTION SIX: LEG EXERCISES

The following exercises target your leg muscles. Your legs are made up of 4 major muscles which are your quadriceps also known as quads which run down the front of your legs, hamstrings which run down the back of your legs, gluteals also known as glutes which are your buttocks muscles and calves which are on the back of your lower leg.

Leg presses and squats target your quads, hamstrings and glutes. Leg extensions target your quads, hamstring curls target your hamstrings. Lunges targets all the leg muscles. Calf raises target your calves.

BARBELL SQUATS

Step 1: Standing at a squat rack place the top of your back under the bar, grip the bar just wider than shoulder width apart and lift the bar off the rack and step back.

Step 2: With your feet facing forward, pointing outward, keep your back arched.

Step 3: Lower yourself down as though you are going to sit on a seat till your thighs are parallel with the floor.

Step 4: Push back through with your legs keeping your feet firmly planted on the floor and keep your back arched, also keep your head up looking up until you are standing upright. Then repeat.

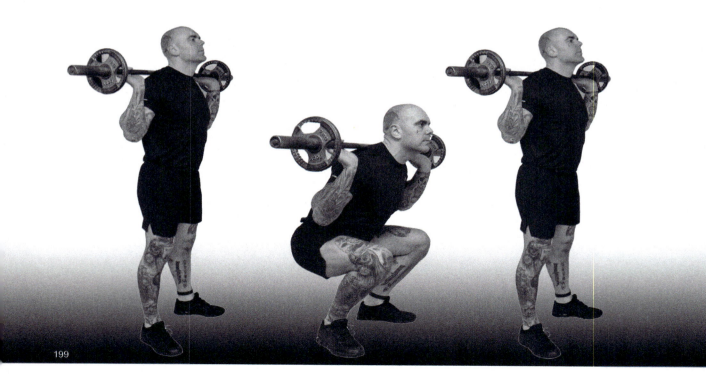

LEG PRESS

Step 1: Sit back on the leg press machine and place your feet shoulder width apart.

Step 2: Lift the weight off and hold the handles.

Step 3: Slowly lower the weight bringing your knees down towards your shoulders keeping your back flat on the seat.

Step 4: Pushing through with your legs push the weight up until your legs are extended. Then repeat.

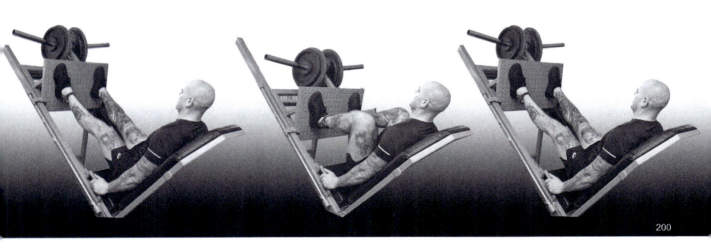

SEATED LEG EXTENSIONS

Step 1: Sitting at the machine place your legs under the pads and adjust the height so the bar is rested on your shins.

Step 2: Keep your back flat on the seat and push through with your quadriceps lifting your feet up until your legs are fully extended in front of you.

Step 3: Lower the weight back down. Then repeat.

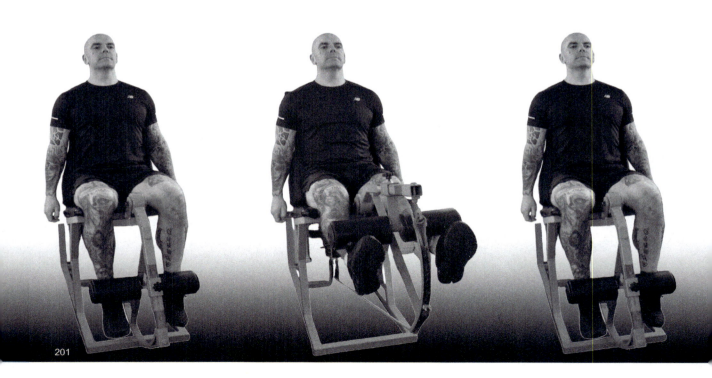

HAMSTRING CURLS

Step 1: Lie on the machine and adjust the setting so the bar is resting at the bottom of your calves.

Step 2: Lift your heels up towards your buttocks and squeeze at the top.

Step 3: Lower the weight back down. Then repeat.

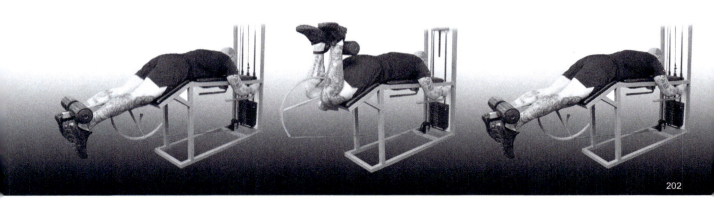

DUMBBELL LUNGES

Step 1: Hold the dumbbells at the side of your legs and stand with your feet hip width apart.

Step 2: Standing upright facing forward place one foot forward.

Step 3: With your leading leg bend forward bending both knees until your rear knee nearly touches the floor, while holding dumbbells at your sides.

Step 4: Push up with your leading leg and step back then repeat on other side.

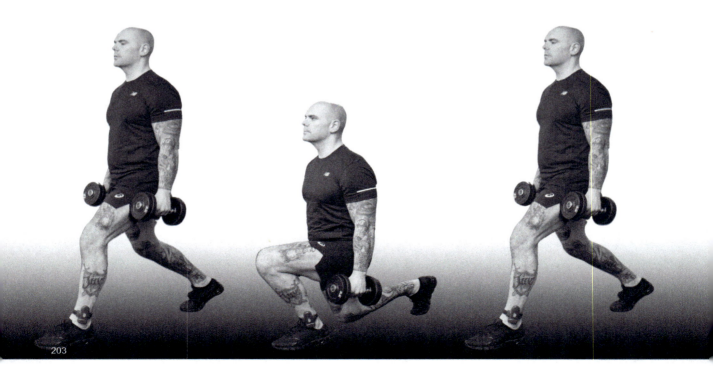

CALF RAISES

Step 1: Place your shoulders under the pads and put the balls of your feet on the stand and push up until you are standing upright with the weight supported on your shoulders.

Step 2: Keeping your legs locked out lower the weight so your heels are lowered towards the floor.

Step 3: Push through with your feet and feel the squeeze in your calves as you go up on the balls of your feet. Then repeat.

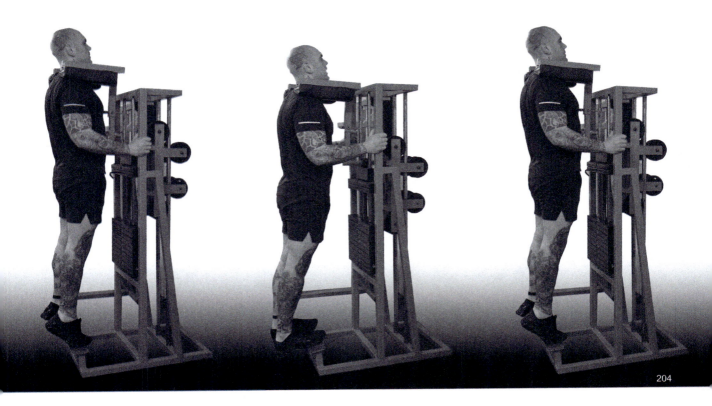

LEG PRESS CALF RAISES

Step 1: Sitting on the machine place the balls of your feet on the plate hip width apart.

Step 2: Lift the weight off and keep your knees slightly bent and your back flat on the machine.

Step 3: Keep your legs extended and just use your ankles to let the weight come back bending your toes backwards so you can feel your calves stretching.

Step 4: Push back through your feet pointing your toes as far forward as you can feeling the squeeze. Then repeat.

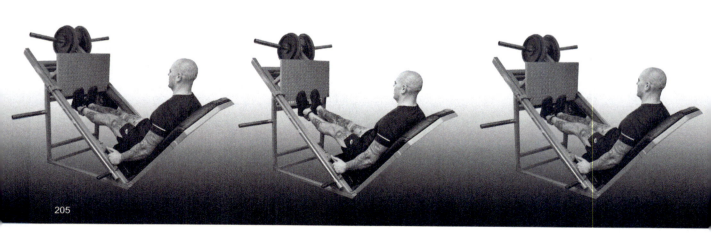

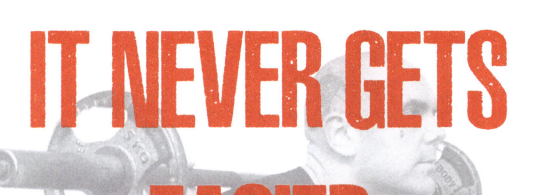

IT NEVER GETS EASIER. YOU ONLY GET BETTER!

ACKNOWLEDGMENTS

First off, I would just like to thank my beautiful wife Mikala for all the love and support she has shown me throughout the 13 months I was locked up and the majority of it 23 hours a day because of the Coronavirus Pandemic.

She has supported me every step of the way and has encouraged me to keep writing this book to help others in this situation.

I was in prison when I was writing this, she has done an incredible job raising our four children on her own.

I would also like to thank my son Ricky who has also continued to workout without me beside him, he is also still doing daily workouts at home and circuits which I have planned for him. At 9 years old he has incredible determination, motivation and he has made me so proud.

I would like to thank my best friend Hopey who has been there for me and my family all the way and has continued to workout out with me on release and we spur each other on, brothers for life.

I would like to thank Becky who I met on the photo shoot for this book coincidentally, as she came along with her friend Kelly to take the photos and we have went on to become friends. She has designed this book for me and put a lot of effort and time into my book.

I would like to thank my friend Stevie Coulson from Stevies Gym for letting me use his gym for the photoshoot for this book.

I would also like to thank Tomma, Celmins, Sasha, Smithy and Nelly from house block 1 in Holme House who I trained with daily and we all supported each other.

I would also like to thank Les The PEI gym officer at Holme House who would come onto the exercise yard throughout the lockdown, workout with us and beast us on some of these circuits. He is one of the fittest blokes I have come across especially for his age 53.

I would also like to thank Rob Dixon, Dean Ward and Singhy who I trained with for the last 5 months on house block 4 in Holme House, keep up the good work lads yous have done well.

Also good luck to the rest of you still serving your sentences and remember don't let a bad situation bring out the worst in you. Be positive and do something good with the rest of your life. Make the rest of your life the best of your life. Good luck.

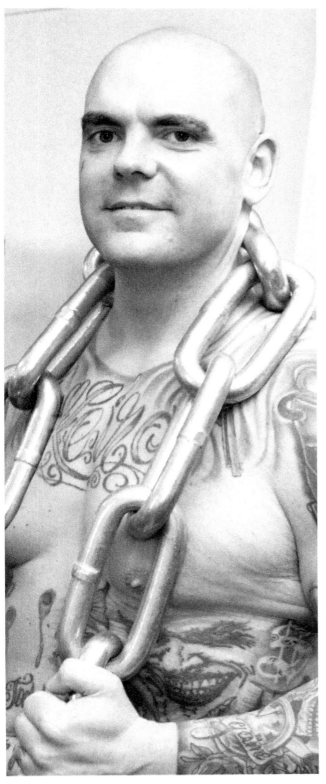

Now I have given you the advice and guidance how to get fitter, stronger, healthier, physically and mentally and how to work out in all areas then if you want to make up your own program then just look through all the different circuits and pick which ones you want to persist with. Use my workout routines and programs until you are fitter and stronger enough to move on to your own routines.

Don't forget, don't get too comfortable with easy workouts or what feels good for you as you will never progress further as it's all about being better than you were yesterday. If your aim is to get as big as possible and as fit as possible, then you should be doing heavyweights as well as bodyweight circuits and I have shown you how to train to do both. So, what you will be doing to achieve this is still following the bulking section of this book but do an additional three bodyweight circuits a week and you will look amazing as your muscles will be getting as big as possible whilst shedding the fat. Ultimately, making you look more bigger and leaner.

If you just want to do weighted circuits in the gym and want to be as lean and as fit as possible whilst maintaining muscle then you will be doing weighted circuits every time you are in the gym, in your back yard or garden with a barbell and you will find this in the barbell circuit sections in this book.

The guidance is there, the rest is up to you and all the help and inspiration is right here. With your own determination and motivation you will soon become an athlete who is fitter, healthier, more focused and positive than ever before. The choice is yours and the beauty of it is you have your own freedom of choice to choose how you want to train, what you want to train, when you want to train and what you want to eat. The world is at your feet, the power is in your hands to want to make that change and make the rest of your life the best of your life. Good luck people and stay strong physically and mentally.

BEFORE & AFTER

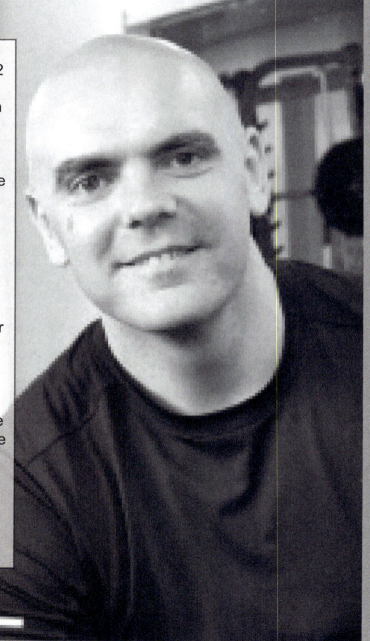

"These are my before and after pictures. What a difference and 2 stone lighter.
So much healthier and fitter both physically and mentally.

Just shows what healthy living and not drinking does. The before pic my head was mashed and was drinking on a regular basis.

Now I feel so fresh and focused. Anyone can do it.
With determination and motivation. I did this on a 23 hour lockdown in the worst place possible.

I made the most out of a bad situation. Went in prison 19 stone with a negative mindset and came out 16 1/2 stone full, of ambition and focusing on the positive things in life. Let go of all the negative shit and life is so much better."
- Ricky Killeen, 2021

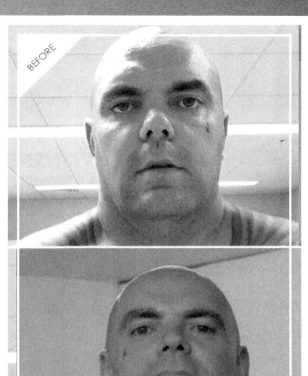
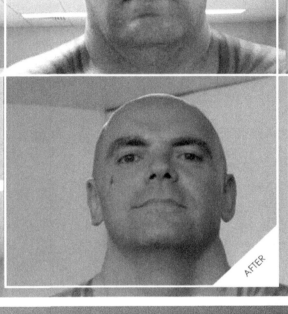
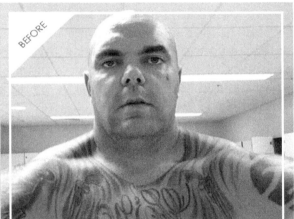
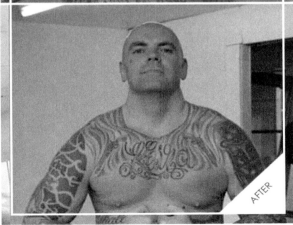

DEDICATION PAGE

I am dedicating this book to the memory of my best friend Toddy (Chris Todd). My best friend since the age of 10, my wife's aunty Linda (Linda Heslin) and my very good friend Ross Hunt. All sadly no longer with us. All who battled with their mental health and thought there was no other way out and sadly took their own lives. Their legacy will live on, may they rest in peace.

I want to try and raise awareness to mental health and let people know its ok to not be ok and its ok to open up and talk about your problems. I'm not saying this book is the answer to people's mental health problems but it will certainly help as it's helped me over the years.

Below is a list of numbers for different charities people can ring if you ever feel there is no way out. There's always light at the end of the tunnel. A simple phone call and a chat can make all the difference.

SAMARITANS 24/7 for prisoners in England and Wales 08457 450 7797

SAMARITANS 24/7 for prisoners in Scotland and N. Ireland 08457 90 90 90

SAMARITANS 24/7 for everybody 116 123

CALM (campaign against living miserably) 5pm-midnight everyday 0800 585858

SOS (silence of suicide) 4pm -midnight 0300 1020 505

MIND (mental health charity) 0300 123 3393

SHOUT crisis text line text "SHOUT" to 85258

IF YOU CARE SHARE foundation 0191 387 5661 (this is a charity in the North East of England that provides suicide prevention, intervention and support for those bereaved by suicide. A local charity of mine that has helped my own friends and family).

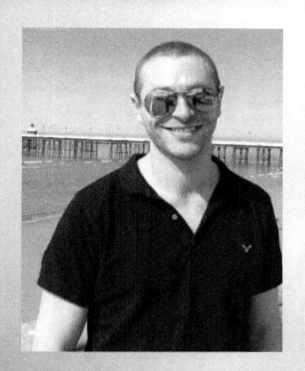
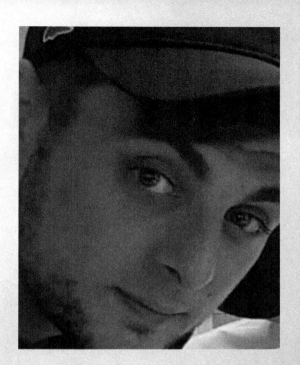
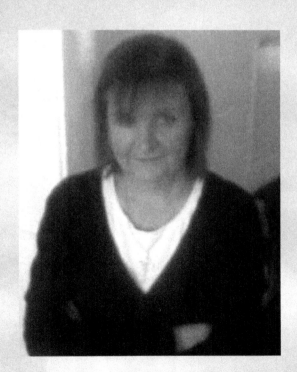

RUTHLESS FITNESS

My trademark: **RUTHLES FITNESS**

This is my trademark which I applied for and was successful. This is the name and logo I am using for my ruthless fitness ventures. I already have a range of clothes available.

All of which can all be found on my website: www.behindthebarsruthlessfitness.co.uk or www.ruthlessfitness.store

Ruthless Fitness

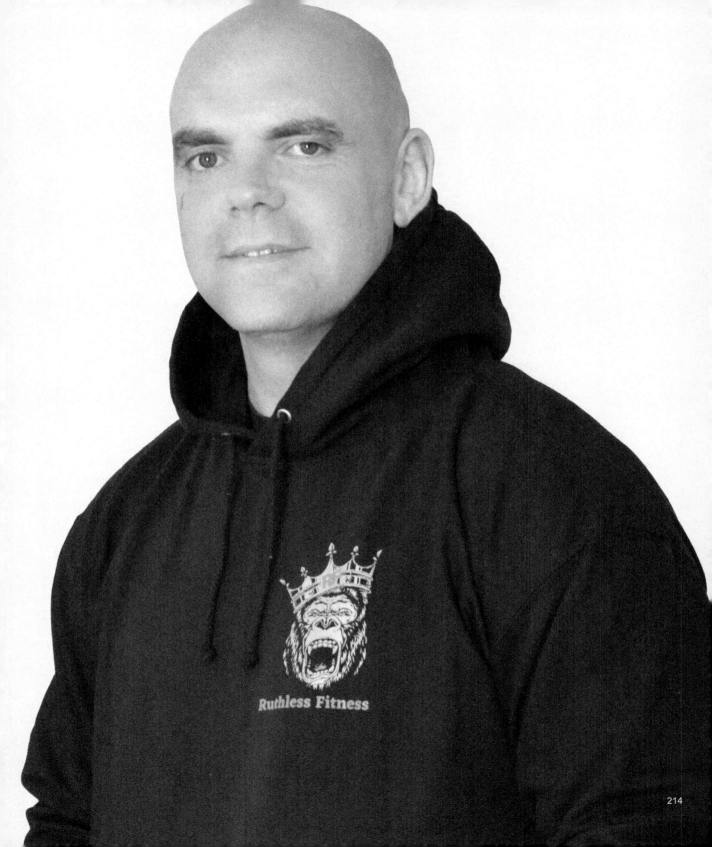

Printed in Great Britain
by Amazon